The
FLYING
NURSE

Saving lives and swaddling babies
from outback Australia to Africa and beyond

The
FLYING
NURSE

Prudence Wheelwright
with Alley Pascoe

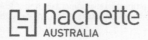
hachette
AUSTRALIA

I would like to acknowledge – and honour – the Traditional Owners of the land on which this book was written and edited: the Arrernte people of the Central Desert Region, the Larrakia people of Darwin and the Gadigal people of the Eora Nation. First Nations sovereignty was never ceded. I pay my respects to Elders past and present and recognise their continuing connection to the land and waters. I thank them for protecting Country since time immemorial.

Note on names and events described in this book: Pseudonyms have been used and other details altered where necessary to protect the identity and privacy of people mentioned.

Content warning: Some parts of this book contain confronting material that might cause distress to some readers.

Published in Australia and New Zealand in 2023
by Hachette Australia
(an imprint of Hachette Australia Pty Limited)
Gadigal Country, Level 17, 207 Kent Street, Sydney, NSW 2000
www.hachette.com.au

Hachette Australia acknowledges and pays our respects to the past, present and future Traditional Owners and Custodians of Country throughout Australia and recognises the continuation of cultural, spiritual and educational practices of Aboriginal and Torres Strait Islander peoples. Our head office is located on the lands of the Gadigal people of the Eora Nation.

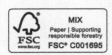 A catalogue record for this work is available from the National Library of Australia

ISBN: 978 0 7336 4884 7 (paperback)

Cover design by Luke Causby, Blue Cork
Photography (front cover) courtesy RFDS; (back cover) courtesy Natalie Stonnill; internal images courtesy author's collection
Typeset in Sabon LT Std by Kirby Jones
Printed and bound in Australia by McPherson's Printing Group

MIX
Paper | Supporting responsible forestry
FSC
www.fsc.org   FSC® C001695

The paper this book is printed on is certified against the Forest Stewardship Council® Standards. McPherson's Printing Group holds FSC® chain of custody certification SA-COC-005379. FSC® promotes environmentally responsible, socially beneficial and economically viable management of the world's forests.

To all who have taught me,
inspired me and continue to love me.
To countless women out there without a voice
and to those who listen.

CONTENTS

PROLOGUE

If there was a colour darker than black, that's what I would use to describe the desert night sky. The darkness is so dense it feels like you could reach out and stroke it. In the pitch blackness of the Northern Territory night, it's impossible to see where the land ends and the sky begins. The horizon doesn't exist.

There's no moon tonight. We only have the stars of the Milky Way and the high beams on this old LandCruiser troopie to guide the way. When I say 'we', I mean Cassie, the Aboriginal health practitioner (AHP), who is driving, and me. I'm sitting in the back seat behind a mother, monitoring her desperately ill three-week-old baby girl strapped into a carrier next to me. On the outside, I'm calm and composed, reassuring the new mum in the front passenger seat as her sick baby chokes for air. In my mind, I'm frantically trying to recall how to resuscitate a three-week-old baby. I flick through the pages of the Standard Treatment Manual of the Central Australian Rural Practitioners Association (CARPA), searching for any advice that might help. I look around the back seat and into the back of the troopie, scoping out space should I need to do a resus. I'm preparing for the worst.

It's my first stint as a remote area nurse (RAN) and midwife – and while this isn't my first emergency trip to the airfield, it's certainly the most serious. This is life and death.

I am one of two nurses; the other is my boss, Karolien, who is currently in Alice Springs on her rostered days off. I often do the same on my days off, so it's usually just one of us on our own in this tiny town in the middle of the desert, three hours drive away from definitive medical care.

I had contacted the Royal Flying Doctor Service (RFDS) for urgent help and we left the clinic in an old LandCruiser and headed straight to the closest airstrip, which is an hour away in the daylight. We don't have the luxury of sunshine.

The darkness makes the already stressful trip all the more desperate.

I am learning that when you do the sort of nursing I'm doing – remote, often solo, having to make decisions that doctors usually make and needing the courage of your convictions – there isn't much room for error. This is one of my first solo emergencies and I am rattled. I want to be better, I want to know more. Tonight, I just want to get this baby to the plane, so she has a chance of staying alive.

Back in the car, navigating the corrugated dirt track, the troopie feels like it's barely holding it together. I know that the young mother in the front seat is barely holding it together. So, I have to hold it together for all of us. That's part of the job, being strong when my patients can't be. And it helps me, too. If I act like I'm in control, it usually has the effect of making me feel in control. Like now. I've never felt more out of control, but you wouldn't know it.

'The plane won't be far away,' I say to nobody in particular, hoping the mother is listening. 'They were going to leave just after I spoke to them.'

What I can't tell her, though, is that her baby will be alright. I don't like to make promises that I can't personally keep, and in this sort of situation all we can do is our best, then we cross our fingers and leave it up to fate, or to God – whatever you choose to believe in. I like to believe in the fundamental decency of human beings and the right of every single person to have adequate healthcare, at the bare minimum. I believe that everyone will feel scared when they're faced with the unknown, and sometimes I represent that unknown, so it's my job not to look away when they feel like that. It's my job to be kind and respectful.

We arrive at the airstrip, and I notice the plane lights circling above. I let out a sigh of relief. The airstrip is drenched in the horizon-hiding darkness. Our first job is to ensure the runway is clear so, horn blaring and high beam on, we speed the distance of the runway to ensure no animals are on the track. A kangaroo jumps out in front of us and Cassie says she'll run it over and chop off its tail to cook over the fire. She's half-joking, I think. I can't be sure, but I'm quietly pleased when the roo bounds into the distance.

When we reach the end of the runway, we turn back and do it again, before parking facing the airstrip and turning the high beam off to let the pilot know that the runway is clear and they're free to land. There is no phone reception out here nor any way of communicating to the pilot or medics on the plane, so we are truly on our own until they land. We wait.

'They'll take care of you,' I say to the newborn, who is still holding on. I wonder if what I have done is enough, if there is anything else I should have done, if she will survive. I need to be better.

The flying doctor plane lands in a rush of air and red dirt. The medics step out onto the runway like they've arrived at this place, to this situation, a hundred times before. This isn't their first rodeo. They're in total control, and I'm in total awe. They've arrived to save the baby, but it also feels like they're saving me from being out of my depth. 'What an incredible job that would be,' I think to myself, watching the RFDS team in their heavy-duty uniforms take over.

When I hand the patient to them, I let out the breath it feels like I've been holding for hours. It's a relief I've never known. It's only after I finish exhaling that I allow myself to feel the magnitude of the situation. Holy shit.

Given the driving conditions and knowing that she doesn't like driving in the dark, I commend Cassie on getting us to the airstrip safely – a miracle in itself – and I take the driver's seat for our hour-long journey home. I make a mental note to send the RFDS my résumé when I'm back in the office. Being a remote area nurse is one thing, but being a rural, flying nurse is another level altogether. I want to be on that level.

First, I must survive the drive home. The darkness leads the way, and our high beams follow.

Crookwell

'Don't sell yourself short because you're a woman.'

– Grandma Mardi

My earliest memory of death is of begging my dad to let me bring a baby lamb home to our farm because its mother had died and I knew it wouldn't survive on its own. Dad said no, he didn't want to take on the responsibility of another animal when the sheep in our paddocks were dying from starvation because of the ongoing drought. At the peak of the drought, we had a mass grave for the sheep we had to destroy, the kinder option than them starving to death. This death pit was an entirely normal part of my childhood.

'It's the cycle of life. We live, and we die,' Dad taught me and my older brother Alex at a very early age.

I come from a long line of Merino sheep farmers, six generations, in fact. My family farm is outside the small town of Crookwell in New South Wales. It's in the Southern Tablelands and the nearest big town is Goulburn. I grew up surrounded by land as far as I could see, often dry in summer and greener in winter. The road to our farm now takes us through a wind farm – it's always a surprise to see how big the white windmills are; they look like something out of a sci-fi movie.

There's a golf club at one end of town and a high school at the other. My primary school was 28 kilometres away from home in an even smaller village called Laggan. It had fifty students, seven of those kids were in my grade: five boys and two girls. In Year Six I was the school captain. We spent our time playing Bull Rush, handball and catch and kiss.

Come high school, my brother Alex and I were sent off to boarding school in Sydney, as was the family tradition. Alex went to The King's School in Parramatta, and I went to Kambala School in Rose Bay, the same as my mother. Kambala was like something out of a storybook. The boarding house balcony had waterfront views overlooking the Sydney Harbour Bridge. Even more interesting to an almost-teenager was the dungeon. Sure, it was solely used to store all the boarders' suitcases, but that didn't make it any less cool to me.

I didn't realise at the time how privileged my brother and I were to go to a boarding school – let alone one with harbour views and a dungeon for storage. I know it wasn't cheap for my parents. Dad, James, ran the farm and Mum, Beth, ran the house and raised two kids. My parents worked ridiculously hard to give us the opportunities that a city education provided. So we went from being outdoor adventure kids in the country covered in mud, climbing trees, swimming in dams and riding motorbikes to being confined to the boarding house rules within a regimented pristine environment.

My brother and I would head straight back to the farm during school holidays, getting our hands dirty and helping Dad. I remember going from a strict school uniform – 'don't forget to wear your hat' – in Sydney to putting on old boots and work clothes and taking some poddy lambs down to Dorrie, a kind-hearted, rough old woman who lived with her pet lambs in a hut with dirt floors. She was completely self-sufficient. Sitting down, drinking tea and making conversation with her was worlds away from the sheer extravagance of visiting my schoolfriends' houses in the eastern suburbs of Sydney.

* * *

Before all of that, we took a family trip to Bali when I was nine. It was my first time overseas and the feeling of stepping off the air-conditioned plane into the tropical Balinese heat has stayed with me ever since. Alex and I spent our time in the massive figure-eight pool eating burgers, while Mum and Dad enjoyed the delicious seafood cuisine. We were too young to appreciate good food. I remember sitting next to Dad on the flight home and staring at the world map on the back of the in-flight magazine in the seat pocket in front of me. Dad asked me if I could point out Bali on the map and, somehow, I found the tiny island in the Indian Ocean. It looked like a speck of dust in comparison to other countries.

Dad and I had one of those lovely end-of-trip chats where we listed our favourite memories from the holiday. There were a few. We'd had a ball.

'Would you like to come back to Bali?' Dad asked me, assuming I'd beg to do it all again on our next holiday.

'No,' I said without hesitation.

He was shocked. 'But why? You really enjoyed it. Why wouldn't you want to go back?'

I just pointed to the world map in front of us. 'Look at all these other places to go,' I said defiantly.

Dad loves telling that story. I don't know if it was because of that moment – or because Dad told the story so many times – but travelling became a core part of my identity. It's all I wanted to do. At school, I didn't know what career I wanted to have, but I knew I wanted to see the world.

When people ask me where I got my sense of adventure from, I say I got it from my grandma. I call her Mardi but Doreen Moore is her actual name. She isn't my biological grandmother; she married my grandfather before I was born, so she's all I've ever known. And how lucky I am to have known her. Mardi was an exceptional woman. She travelled the world in the 1960s with her work as a physiotherapist, spending most of her career in Canada to then become head of the World Confederation for Physical Therapy, holding global physiotherapy conferences around the world, including at the Sydney Opera House in 1987, which was at the time the largest and most comprehensive gathering of physiotherapists ever held. All in a very male-dominated field.

She was strong, altruistic, worldly and authoritative. With an innate belief in change for the better, she was a trailblazer in the physiotherapy world. She was a fearless woman.

When Mardi's mum fell ill, she came home to Australia, where she was reacquainted with my grandpa at age forty-seven and went on to marry him. That's how my family came to be blessed with the independent spirit of our Mardi. She didn't have children of her own, so she passed down her wisdom to me, my brother and my cousins. Mardi was all about women's education and empowerment and she taught me that I could be anything I wanted to be – just like she had. The stories of her adventures gallivanting around the globe stirred something deep inside me.

While Mardi was perhaps the greatest influence on my sense of adventure, if you ask my mum she'll say that I was so adventurous as a child that they had to put barbed wire on top of the fence to stop me getting out! She'd also say that whenever they couldn't find me they'd know I'd be up a tree somewhere. I have always been a risk taker. I'd climb the tallest branch in the highest tree, then ask myself, *How do I get down?* Then the branch would break and I'd fall! My parents didn't try to stop me; they just let me go and figure things out for myself.

One time we were on our way to visit my grandparents in Walgett when we stopped in at cattleyards in Dubbo. I was dressed in my Sunday best, but that didn't stop me hopping up on the catwalk that hovered above the cattle pens. Next thing my parents knew, I'd managed to swing myself downwards and accidentally slip down the rails into a cattle-filled pen of wet cow manure. An unknown man plucked me out so I didn't get trampled, but it wasn't quickly enough to stop me getting covered in cow shit. Regretting the clothing choice she'd made for me, Mum took me to a cramped, cold public toilet to wash the cow faeces out of my long blonde hair.

The adventurous instinct extends to my brother, Alex: he used to travel as much as I do, and there was one time when we were together and told Mum that we'd be out of touch for three days because we were going to explore the Corn Islands in Nicaragua, where there was no reception. By the sixth day of no contact our parents were convinced we were dead. We were, in fact, completely safe, drinking Flor de Caña rum and eating lobster. When we were finally able to get off the island and send them a message, it was to let them know that there'd been a storm and we hadn't been able to get off the island any sooner. Obviously that was a little too much adventure for them, but it never stopped us.

It could be in our blood: my father has a book about the Wheelwright family, which has a centuries-old history of travelling the globe and undertaking adventures. According to this book, my ancestors include entrepreneurs, explorers, eccentrics, philosophers, scientists, soldiers and sailors as well as artists, doctors and diplomats. One was a sea captain who became a pirate; another was a lawyer who became a globe-trotting sportsman.

At some point in my childhood, one of Mardi's equally fabulous friends from America came to visit us in Australia. Her name was Sue Adler and she was a pilot. Over a meal of Mum's infamous roast lamb with all the trimmings, when Sue asked me what I wanted to do with my life, I told her I was thinking about being an air hostess.

'Absolutely not,' she said, slamming a glass down on the table for effect. 'You will not be an air hostess, you'll be the pilot. None of this sitting down the back of the plane serving sandwiches, you'll be in the front seat flying the plane.'

With Sue's words and Mardi's legacy guiding me, I vowed never to sell myself short because I was a woman. And I hoped to live a life half as exciting as theirs.

* * *

I never set out to be a nurse. I didn't dream about wearing scrubs and emptying bedpans as a little girl, nor did I have nursing on my wish list of careers in high school. I had no family members in the field, nor a selfless devotion for helping people.

Some people say that nursing is their calling. For me, it was a bargaining chip. After I left school, I had no career aspirations, but I knew I wanted to take a gap year to travel. So, it was agreed, I would scratch my travel bug overseas and then I'd come back to Australia and get a degree – in what didn't matter, I just had to get one. My parents insisted.

I applied for an organised gap year program in London and requested an 'outdoor activities' placement. My request was denied, but I was accepted for a carer's role. As a selfish teenager, I wasn't thrilled with the idea of having to look after other people. But the placement gave me a ticket to the other side of the world for a year, so away I went.

Arriving in England as a relatively sheltered eighteen-year-old and being placed in a nursing home for severely disabled adults was a shock. There were women with spina bifida who spent their days bent in half, car accident victims who were physically there but not mentally, and people born with no limbs due to genetic abnormalities. The clients were unable to care for themselves. They needed assistance for all daily activities, from eating to walking, rolling over and toileting. I was that assistance.

For the first two months at the nursing home, I wanted to run away. It was all too confronting: the screams, the responsibility, the unescapable smell of disinfectant. I didn't think I was cut out for it. But with a stern talking to from my family, and memorable life chat along the lines of: 'In life you have to give things time to adjust, so give it your all and if in three months you are still unhappy then we can look at moving you', I was just as surprised as anyone when three months rolled around and I came to love the job, the patients and everything in between. There was something so satisfying about making people smile when smiling seemed impossible. By this time too, I'd met my friend Andy, who worked within the same organisation and lived nearby in a house full of young people who all became my saving grace.

I came out of my six-month placement feeling pretty chuffed with myself, but mostly just excited to spend the next six months travelling. I was still a teenager, after all. I had no idea that my time at the nursing home would go on to shape the rest of my life.

Later I was working on a farm in the snow-dusted Yorkshire Dales through a family connection, hammering staples to fence posts, when I called home to check in.

'It's time to apply for university admissions,' my mother said.

'I don't think I'll come back,' I said, testing my luck.

'You have to, Prue. It's what we agreed.'

My mother is a kind-hearted woman, but she didn't raise us kids by being soft on us, so I can't say her response was a surprise. I'd hoped she'd maybe let me off the hook. Not that I'm her favourite child or anything – she doesn't have one, apparently – but don't we all hope that we'll be let off the hook sometime?

'I was thinking that maybe I could apply next year ...' I said, hoping to buy time while I worked out a rationale.

'Prudence,' my mother warned in the tone that told me there was no point fighting.

'Okay,' I said, capitulating. 'Just put me down for whatever you like. But what I really want is to keep doing this. I want to travel. So could you choose something that helps me do this again?'

Cheeky, wasn't I? Asking my mum to be my personal assistant and fill in my admission forms.

Mum's non-negotiable attitude to our education stemmed from her own experience. She regretted never furthering her education after high school – like me, she had so much fun as a young adult just out of school with a fantastic social life that she never pursued a tertiary education, and her parents didn't insist on it. She was adamant about my brother and I going to university, something I will forever be grateful for.

A week or so later, Mum called and told me she had enrolled me in nursing and teaching degrees. I said, disheartened, 'I don't want to be a teacher – that sounds horrible! And a nurse, Mum? Hell no!'

I had to change my attitude when I was accepted into a combined nursing/teaching degree at Charles Sturt University in Bathurst, which was probably what I deserved, given that I asked her to choose.

Before I headed to uni, I had the time of my life in Europe, doing the obligatory Contiki trip as a nineteen-year-old, spending more time drinking than revelling in the glorious scenery and history. I went to Greece with Laura, my good friend to this day, with a budget of 10 euros a day. The day I was put in charge of food I brought home watermelon, bread and spam – I've never been forgiven for this. I also had a white Christmas in Norway with Henriette, my lifelong friend I met in boarding school, and her family. Coming home was a bit of a shock!

Fortunately my brother and friend Alex was at the same university so the transition to campus life and making friends was easy. It was here I first met my brother's good mate James, and was told sternly by Alex that he was 'off limits', which of course only made me want him more. James, in turn, was told by Alex to stay away from me.

I found studying at university pretty hard. I had been terrible at schoolwork, and I was terrible at university work. How I got through any of it is a miracle. I have only realised in the last few years that I'm a visual learner, a practical learner. I am much better at the practical side of things, and touching. I'm a tactical learner. Knowing that now, I can actually formulate how I learn, rather than being in a classroom and reading something and then retaining it and writing an essay. I still find that so hard.

Growing up in a small community, we had to adapt to talking to all age groups and personalities. I was used to talking to elderly people one minute, then having chats with toddlers the next.

So for me, university was more social and fun than educational and academic. I worked three jobs, saved money and spent university holidays overseas. Most importantly, I made a lifelong friend, Claire, who was doing the same degree as me, and we helped each other through. Mostly by deciding to watch *Grey's Anatomy* instead of going to class. After all, it's about medicine ...

Initially I'd thought, 'I love kids. I'll go down the childcare road and just do the nursing because I got into it.' But after a year of writing thousand-word essays about why babies roll over – what more can you say other than 'it's a developmental stage'? – I realised that early childhood education was not for me.

I wasn't that fussed on nursing, either, until I went to a presentation from a visiting lecturer. Sitting in a lecture hall, a photo appeared on the slideshow that immediately captured my attention. The photos were from Médecins Sans Frontières (MSF) – the legendary medical humanitarian organisation which helps people affected by conflicts, disasters and diseases the world over. The first photo was of nurses working in a dusty field in a tent somewhere with minimal equipment. The next showed an infamous image of a famine-ravaged child in Ethiopia, bent over with a vulture lurking in the background. This photo was so much more than a slide in a presentation to me – it was the spark that lit a fire inside me. The lecturer showed me that nursing wasn't just hospital shiftwork – it could open up the world.

'This is what I want to do,' I thought to myself. 'I want to work for MSF one day.'

A dream was born.

Thanks to my very full social life, it took me four years instead of the standard three to finish my degree. Within this time the forbidden fruit, James, and I were in a committed relationship, living together off campus and enjoying being young and in love. I adored him for his humour, his mannerisms and his patience and understanding of me; he was my person. We couldn't go more than three days without seeing each other. We were completely infatuated.

When I finally finished university, I was lucky to be accepted at Royal Prince Alfred Hospital in Sydney, which meant I went straight into a big tertiary teaching hospital. This was the bee's-knees of jobs for new graduates because the hospital was, and is, so dedicated to teaching. James stayed behind in Bathurst to work and came to Sydney to see me most weekends. Committing to a long-distance relationship was the beginning of our undoing.

I settled in to work at RPA quickly, making friends, living in shared housing and enjoying a busy social life. I worked for two years rotating around the renal, gastro, medical and surgical wards – a bit of everything. James and I saw each other whenever we could. Then I decided to study midwifery. It was a totally different approach to medicine, and I had developed an interest in women's health.

My year of midwifery studies was hellish, from university work and RPA-specific assignments to recording a portfolio of every interaction with a pregnant woman. My social life and relationships suffered. While I made it through, my relationship of six years with James sadly did not.

I got my registration, only to be advised as soon as I finished that I should do postgraduate studies straight away 'to consolidate all the skills you've learned'. My lecturers, colleagues and parents pushed for me to stay on the right path, to focus on my career, to stick to the status quo.

Instead, newly single and itching to scratch the travel bug, I bought a one-way ticket to Cape Town in South Africa and hopped on a plane. I didn't have a return ticket or any plans to go home. The only plan I had was to head north on that vast continent. I didn't look back.

It wasn't the first, or last, time I'd take a leap into the unknown.

Arriving in Cape Town, I quickly realised I was quite vulnerable as a lone female traveller, so I got online and managed to book overland travel trips for a quarter of the price, leaving the next day. I joined a truck for three weeks with twelve others to head to the Zambezi. This is how I travelled north over the next eight months, jumping on and off tours and doing a bit of solo travel in between. In the process I sat among gorillas in giant stinging nettles in Rwanda, watched humpbacks breach off the coast of Mozambique, climbed epic sand dunes in Namibia, ate deep-fried insects in Botswana and bungee-jumped 111 metres into Victoria Falls in Zimbabwe. I sat in awe at the Valley of the Kings in Egypt, drank cocktails and danced in Zanzibar, hot-air ballooned above the Serengeti, saw 'the big five' and walked among graceful giraffes. I could keep going – I have so many wonderful memories from this trip. I had a beautiful, mind-blowing love affair lasting many months across multiple countries and made lifelong friends along the way. It really was the trip of a lifetime and only added to my desire to travel and live and work overseas. Africa seemed to have a soul and rhythm below the surface. I fell in love with the continent. To work here with MSF was still my dream.

Of course, travelling cost money and I was running out, so it was time to go home – but not before an impromptu trip to America with a ticket my good friends Tarz and Jess had offered me to join them at Burning Man, a world-renowned eight-day festival in the Nevada Desert famous for its leave-no-trace attitude.

After that, I was ready to go home and needed to work. But on arriving home and seeing my family, eating the infamous roast lamb dinner cooked by Mum and catching up with friends, the travel itch was still raging. So I applied for a job in Saudi Arabia, combining my love of travel and work and adventure into the unknown.

CHAPTER ONE

Riyadh, Saudi Arabia

*'Welcome to a sweet jail. It is sweet because you
earn money, it is jail as you don't find much
happiness here.'*

– Wahid, my driver

It started the same way all my adventures do, with five
words written in a brand-new diary: 'And so it begins
again ...'

I landed in Saudi Arabia – after eighteen hours of
travelling – as the sun was rising. The light of day ripped
the curtains open and awakened the sleeping city of Riyadh.
I knew nothing about Saudi except its reputation. The
kingdom has long restricted political rights and personal

freedoms, especially the civil liberties of women, who, at the time I was there, were banned from driving, drinking alcohol and interacting with men they're not related to. The gender division was immediately apparent when we landed at the airport and women and men were separated into different areas to be patted down by security.

'Why would you want to spend a year living somewhere like that?' you might ask. You're not alone. I asked myself that very question when I chose to head to Saudi over staying in my happy and safe life in Australia. After eight months of adventure travelling through Africa, being home just wasn't an option for me. I wanted to experience something different, somewhere off the mainstream track and out of the ordinary. I wanted to chase the unknown.

I was intrigued by Saudi Arabia because of its perception in the West. I wanted to see it for myself. I figured it couldn't be as bad as people made out. There had to be some good in the place, and I wanted to find it. At the time, you couldn't visit Saudi Arabia as a tourist, it was a locked country, which meant you had to have a job organised before you could even enter the country. What's behind the closed door? That's exactly what I set out to find when I joined an agency as a registered nurse and accepted a twelve-month placement at the King Faisal Specialist Hospital and Research Centre in the capital city of Riyadh.

Riyadh has a population of more than seven million, and it's built on a desert plateau in the middle of the country. It is a city of stark contrasts. The historic district of Deira stands in the shadow of the modern Kingdom skyscraper, which is one of the most iconic buildings, and the subject of many discussions in the expat community. Depending on who you ask, the tower is either the shape of a burqa – in a country that doesn't have a lot of female representation – or in the shape of a bottle opener – in a country where alcohol is forbidden.

The roads are pure chaos, with the street rules of a developing country, but they're lined with designer shops: Cartier, Ferrari and Chanel. The infamous Chop Chop Square – where public executions, usually beheadings, took place each Thursday – is a children's playground every other day of the week. In the middle of the square's well-manicured courtyard is a drain. One day that drain is covered in blood; the next day kids are riding their scooters over it. Time stands still, but also rushes past.

I didn't have much time to explore my new city before I started the orientation process at the hospital. The building is all sharp angles and reflective windows that mirror back the lush gardens outside, including palm trees and fountains. Inside, the ceilings are unexpectedly low. If I jumped, I would have hit my head – and I'm a short-arse. I didn't jump. On my first day, I learned that the royal family has its own hospital wing, and that's where I was assigned to work. It's more like a hotel than a hospital. You enter the ward via a gold lift!

Because there are no disability homes or rehabilitation centres in Saudi, any members of the royal family who are born with congenital issues or disabilities, or who are paralysed because of a car accident or the like, live on this ward. The ward is staffed by international workers, and each patient has their own 'sitter', a personal support worker – predominantly from the Philippines – who lives in the room with them, feeds them, bathes them and provides all their daily care. The nurses, on the other hand, are tasked with giving out medication.

This would be the extent of my role, I came to learn. There was a lot to learn. One lesson that was drilled into the new nurses: 'Forget everything you know, be a student again, shut up and listen.' I heard it so many times a day, I started to tune out – in total opposition of the last command. Oops.

During my orientation at the hospital, I was fitted for my all-white uniform, which included a lab coat. It was all very official – and quite exciting. So, too, was buying my first abaya at the Dira Souk, an open-air marketplace. I picked out a beautiful black abaya for AU$34 and another cheaper option for AU$21.

An abaya is different to a burqa. The abaya is a long robe or cloak that is worn over clothes and tends to cover the whole body from the neck to the hands and down to the feet. It's paired with a head scarf or hijab to cover the hair. The burqa, similarly, is a garment that covers the whole body and face. They both serve as a symbol of modesty, privacy and morality.

I thought I might feel suffocated wearing an abaya, but there's something liberating about it; not having to worry about what you look like, or what you're wearing (or not wearing) underneath, or how people see you. It was an unusual – and unexpected – feeling.

I must admit when I first arrived and saw groups of women wearing abayas, it was confronting and intimidating. Now, putting one on has made me realise that we're all people underneath and it's not intimidating at all, more a feeling of community and belonging. In my conversations with local women, they told me about the positives of wearing an abaya. For them, it's not a matter of being controlled, it's a choice they make. They choose to be a part of their community.

I was in the honeymoon phase of culture shock where everything seems new and exciting. I knew this high would be followed by a low of loneliness and isolation. It was coming, I just didn't know when. I wasn't going to sit around and wait for it, though. Fortunately, I got an invite from a colleague to the Canadian Embassy for a game of hockey (using ice hockey sticks with a puck on a tennis court) and a gin (for the bargain price of $2.50 a drink). I was one of a handful of Aussies, among Kiwis, Canadians, Brits, Filipinos, Yanks and some very friendly Irish. There was a barbeque cooking, a guitar playing, drinks flowing and laughter roaring. It was like hanging out in a mate's backyard in Australia. It certainly didn't feel like I was in Saudi Arabia. But reality hit as I got ready to leave. I put on my abaya and hijab, went through security and signed myself out of the embassy before I stepped outside. I was fully covered sitting up straight in the back of a taxi and looking outside at a dust storm rolling in. Also, I was pretty tipsy.

I soon acquired a personal driver whose name was Wahid. He came recommended by a fellow nurse I'd met and soon we became friends. I trusted him. He drove me wherever I needed to go and when he was unavailable, he would send someone else to collect me. I remember one day after an embassy party I was in a formal, floor-length red dress and somehow, after having too much to drink, found myself somewhere unknown and unsafe out on the street without my abaya. I called Wahid in a panic describing what I could see, and he came to find me and take me home to safety. Having a driver was normal and necessary for women and also common for men, being cheaper and more convenient than owning a car.

I lived in an apartment in an expat compound, Complex C, Room 504, which I had to myself. The complex had a pool, internet lab, laundry room, pool table, spa and a book swap. The corridors were long and empty – quite different to the corridors of the hospital.

On my first day of work after orientation, I realised within the first few hours that my job was less about nursing and more about jumping as high as the patients wanted me to; doing what they wanted, when they wanted, how they wanted. There were sixteen long-term patients on my ward, and they all had routines that us nurses needed to work around. It's a different way of working – and there's a different way of thinking, too.

There are entire wards in the Middle East dedicated to the preservation of patients in a vegetative state, who believe that it's Allah's will, *inshallah*. Locals in Saudi don't pay for healthcare, so they don't have to consider the amount it costs to preserve the life of someone who is brain dead. I saw a young baby hooked up to an extracorporeal membrane oxygenation (ECMO) machine. This machine pumps blood outside of your body to a heart-lung machine that removes carbon dioxide and sends oxygen-filled blood back to tissues in the body. I thought about what might lie ahead for her. What's the point of living if there's zero quality of life? It's not a question that's considered in Saudi. There's a belief that if life can be sustained, it should be. All I saw was a dying patient, who was unable to die. It's invasive and cruel, and it's all for nothing. The person is going to die. We can only delay the inevitable for so long. Their way of thinking was hard for me to understand, but it's not my place to cast judgement.

In that hospital I wasn't sure what my place was exactly, but it certainly was not nursing. At work I felt more like a glorified babysitter than a registered nurse and midwife. In a twelve-hour shift, I could go all day without seeing two of my four patients, because they didn't like being disturbed. When I tried to check in on them, their hired staff told me that they were fine. Once I had a tissue box thrown at me.

'How do you know they are fine?' I asked.

'Oh, we do obs on them,' they would say.

That might be well and good, but what were the observations, were they within normal limits, was the patient in pain, did they need analgesia? There was documentation to be done and this was very hard to do when you had not seen the patient. Most days I simply wrote: 'Patient refusing to see nurse today, sitters ensure patient is well.'

Like Riyadh itself, my days were filled with stark contrasts. I had a gorgeous elderly patient recovering from knee surgery who smiled at me, called me beautiful and filled my pockets with chocolates. Then I had a long-term patient who was dependent on oxycodone, but instead of treating her addiction, we were expected to fuel it by giving her the medication she was hooked on. It was infuriating. There are no rehab centres, nursing homes, disability services or palliative care wards in Saudi. For such a rich country, the lack of health resources is shocking.

After work, I felt like a stiff drink, but that isn't an option. The only place where drinking is allowed – or overlooked – is at the foreign embassies, because they're considered foreign soil so the Saudi rules don't apply. Even though the embassies offer a reprieve from the rules, the gatherings are regimented rather than spontaneous. To get into an embassy, you need to have someone put your name on a list and to sign you in and out. You also need to pass three or four checkpoints where armed soldiers pat you down and x-ray scan you.

Not all embassies are made the same. I started to learn which ones had real drinks – Corona, Bombay Sapphire Gin and decent wine – and which ones served homebrew moonshine, called *sid*. The latter is potent, and infamous in the expat community. You can have a cracking night on the moonshine or a total disaster – there's no in-between, and you never know which way it will go.

There's an urgency to the partying in Saudi. Once in a blue moon when an embassy threw a party, our phones would be put in envelopes prior to the event and stacked away until we signed out. There were no photos allowed and we had to pass through a security check. Eventually we'd enter these extravagant balls, dressed to the nines in formal wear, and line up at the bar for a drink, then sit down for three-course meals. The events would be on a time limit so we had just four and a half hours to have a few drinks, eat in style, and let loose to have some autonomy over our lives. Then it was back to abayas, segregation and sobriety.

I turned twenty-seven three weeks after landing in Saudi Arabia. It was a birthday unlike any I'd had before. When I called an Italian restaurant to make a booking for my birthday dinner, the waiter made a pre-emptive apology. 'I'm sorry, the staff won't be able to sing "Happy Birthday" to you or put up any celebration signs,' he said. 'Our branch has been warned by the Mutawa (also known as the Islamic religious police) not to hold any birthday parties. Our manager just got out of jail after a few nights there,' he explained matter-of-factly.

'Um, right, okay,' I replied, not exactly expecting a happy birthday song or signs, but it was weird to be told you can't have those things. I didn't quite know what to expect, but the waiter was happy to take my booking and didn't seem worried about their operating conditions since it was just a dinner, not a birthday outing.

So, there was no alcohol to toast with, no singing, or cake to cut, but there was good company and tasty bruschetta. It was all very civilised, unlike other birthdays where I've ended up dancing on tables and sleeping underneath them. The night was women-only and defined by many rules but there were no issues and I went home happy.

On my way home from the restaurant, I opened the door of the car to find a beautiful bunch of flowers from Wahid. It was a sweet gesture from a kind man, who became my friend and unofficial tutor in Middle Eastern life. He was from Pakistan and was working in Saudi to provide for his family back home. When I first got to Saudi, Wahid had welcomed me to the country and described it as a 'sweet jail'. It certainly felt like that sometimes.

Nothing is easy in Saudi. To get internet access, you need to already have internet access to sign up. To get a SIM card for a mobile, you need an Iqama number to prove you're a resident. To leave the country (after your first three months of passportlessness), you need to apply for a Saudi visa and wait four weeks for it to be processed. Even ducking to the shops to get a box of cereal isn't a simple task, which is something I learned the hard way … The first time it happened, I was standing in the cereal aisle deciding between frosted flakes or sultana bran when the doors closed and the shop came to a complete halt. For a second, I wondered if there was an emergency or a robbery taking place. The staff at the counters stopped working and everyone in the store dropped to their hands and knees facing toward Mecca. It was prayer time, which happens five times a day and waits for no cereal craving. All you can do is politely wait until the doors are open, the till beeps and the store starts operating again like nothing has happened.

* * *

My first acute case in the royal ward was a young prince with a kicked toe. He demanded a CT scan, which was totally unnecessary, but the doctors obliged and organised one. I wanted to tell him that he didn't need anything – he'd just stubbed his toe! – but instead I took his blood pressure, gave him paracetamol and set him up in his royal suite.

After he'd settled in, one of his staff approached me and gave me an envelope containing US$500.

'Whoa, we don't accept money from patients,' was my first thought. I also couldn't help wondering if he was expecting something else in return for his five hundred bucks.

I immediately went to see my supervisor. 'The prince gave me money!' I said, showing her the envelope, expecting her to be as shocked as I was.

Instead, she shrugged. 'It's a tip. You can keep it.'

I didn't want to – it was totally against all my training and the nursing culture I knew. But there was no way to give it back without causing insult.

My first tip was closely followed by my second. It came from a princess who was literally served her tablets individually on a silver spoon. She was, however, trumped by another princess who requested an IV so all her medication could be given intravenously. She couldn't possibly swallow a pill!

* * *

The honeymoon phase was over. I was struggling to find purpose in my job there, and I felt like I was losing all the nursing skills I'd worked so hard to gain. I made the call to leave the royals (and their tips) behind to move downstairs to the public surgical ward. The work would be harder and more intense, but I've never been afraid of hard work. I was a nurse, not a babysitter.

When they say, 'Be careful what you wish for', they're talking about the surgical ward at King Faisal Specialist Hospital and Research Centre. Even though they were in the same hospital, the royal and surgical wards were worlds apart. I had expected a bigger workload and more pressure than what I had been under, but nothing could have prepared me for the total chaos of the surgery department. Unlike the royal ward where I had four patients a shift to look after, there was no nurse–patient ratio in the surgical ward. I worked twelve-hour shifts and was running the whole time.

In Saudi Arabia they performed HIPEC (hyperthermic intraperitoneal chemotherapy) surgeries, which were not done in Australia at that time. To treat an abdominal cancer, they open up the patient and keep them propped open with a retractor contraption, then cut out all the cancer. After that they pump hot chemotherapy liquid into the abdominal cavity, leave it there for twenty minutes or so to kill any bad cells, and pump it back out again before replacing the organs and sewing up the patient.

This is a controversial, and risky, surgery which requires a lot of post-operative nursing care, including the use of epidurals – usually only given to women in labour – and us nurses looked after five or six of these patients at once. I looked after a patient who was still in hospital sixteen days after her HIPEC surgery. She had a vacuum-assisted closure on her wound, which the hospital staff wanted to remove so they could send her home. Their plan was to stick the wound together with surgical glue and sterile strips. It was a recipe for an infection. I advocated for the patient and bought her one more day in the hospital. The next day, the fight would start again.

It was exhausting and hard work, but the staff from every corner of the world brought with them their own set of skills and stories, so work was always intriguing and interesting; just dealing with language barriers alone was a full-time job. Dealing with the bureaucracy and paperwork was another full-time job, and somehow we had to squeeze some nursing in between it all.

The bureaucracy didn't end at work. Two of my friends – fellow nurses – were arrested for being in the company of a man. They had been watching a football match at the house of the ward clerk – a local Saudi man – when the Mutawa smashed through the front door. Someone must have dobbed them in. The women were chucked into the back of a van, kicking and screaming, and taken to the police station. There, they were strip-searched. They were imprisoned for two nights and had their passports confiscated for three months, leaving them trapped in the country.

The whole ordeal was wild, but what I found even wilder was how desensitised everyone was about it. There was sympathy, but not a huge amount of shock. It was as though two young women being thrown in jail for watching a football match with a bloke was normal.

James, my ex, was in a committed relationship by this point, but I found myself pining for him. I missed him and somehow made this wild fantasy in my brain that we would be together again one day. I was lonely. But simply knowing he was in the world made things okay. Therefore, wherever I was in the world, I was okay. A fantasy was born.

I started to feel the walls closing in. For someone like me who gets itchy feet from standing in the same spot for too long, it was suffocating. Travel is my escape. When I chose to spend a year in Saudi, I did so because I wanted to explore the unknown, but also because I wanted to explore all the countries around the unknown. Saudi is conveniently situated a short flight away from Sri Lanka, Jordan, Thailand, Burma, Dubai, Oman, Bahrain, Qatar, Spain, Portugal and Singapore; and a slightly longer flight away from London, New York, Canada and Norway. I made travel plans for all of them by rigging my hospital roster so I worked seven days in a row, had five days off and booked in an extra two days of annual leave on top of that, so it was one week on, one week off. In my bedroom, I dedicated an entire wall to my travel plans, sticking up flight confirmations, accommodation options and to-do lists.

On the plane trip back from my first escape to Sri Lanka, most of the passengers were wearing comfy tracksuits and casually lounging around in their seats and in the aisles. When the captain announced we'd crossed over into Saudi airspace, it was like a switch was flicked. The women stood up and shuffled into their abayas. They sat up straight with their hands in their laps for the rest of the journey. Just like that, we were back in Saudi before we had even landed. Welcome back to 'sweet jail'.

When I returned to work, I walked into the women's bathroom and was welcomed by a friendly person who seemed to know I had been away. She said that the ward had missed me. Totally muddled as to who this person was, I went along with it until eventually I had to ask, 'I'm sorry, do I know you?' The woman laughed and pulled up her burqa to show her eyes, and the penny dropped. It was Mirium, a graceful doctor I'd worked daily with but whose face I had never seen.

On days when I felt crushed by the rigidity of Saudi, I stared at my travel wall. I also carried out little acts of rebellion ... When I was going between the accommodation compounds or out to the shops, I put my abaya on and nothing else. I was fully covered, but also starkers. It was a silly way of reclaiming autonomy, but it kept me sane.

I spent that year travelling, adapting and falling in love with all opportunity that came my way. What brings people together the world over is food, music, sport, kindness and family. In Saudi I found all of this and made lifelong friends along the way. Alas the year with all its international travel opportunities was coming to an end. After farewell wishes and final goodbyes I took my final plane trip out of Riyadh, a year well spent.

CHAPTER TWO

Central Australia

'If you see the Todd River flow three times, that makes you a local.'

– Alice Springs folklore

Ibrought my abaya home with me. It's a reminder of my time in Saudi Arabia and of the stark contrast between cultures. It was also an interesting topic of conversation for my family and friends, who asked me to try it on for them and then marvelled, 'I don't know how you wore that for an entire year!' I felt unexpectedly defensive of Saudi. When people asked me questions about my time there, they didn't really listen to my answers. Instead, they latched on to their preconceived notions of the place and used my stories to solidify those notions. I tried to explain how beautiful the culture was, how kind the people were and what the reality was like for women in the region, but all they heard was burqas, public beatings and alcohol bans. It was frustrating.

Arriving back in Australia from Saudi Arabia was a sort of reverse culture shock. Going from such a huge concrete city to the lush greenery of the east coast gave me whiplash. I was home, but I didn't know where I belonged anymore. I knew for sure I couldn't go back to Sydney to work again. I'd done my time in the city, and while I enjoyed it and am grateful for all that it taught me in life and work, it's not for me.

'Where to next?' I wondered, but not for long. My good friends, Nik and Junitta, whom I met in my first year as a nurse at RPA, were living in Alice Springs and invited me out there. I'd never been to the Northern Territory, and that's all I needed to pique my interest. I applied for a job at the local hospital and got it. Then I hit the road.

To NT locals, the Stuart Highway is known as 'The Track'. As tracks go, it's a pretty long one: 2711 kilometres of straight bitumen that runs from Port Augusta in South Australia all the way up to Darwin at the Top End. The speed limit on the highway is 20 kilometres faster than everywhere else in the country. The 130 kilometres per hour speed sign told me that I was a long way from home. So, too, did the stickiness of the bitumen under the ruthless outback sun.

Arriving in Alice Springs after five days on the road, the first thing I noticed was how the MacDonnell Ranges hug the town and welcome visitors from the south; Heavitree Gap is like an open gate between the East and West Ranges, with the usually dry Todd River flowing through the middle.

On any given day at Alice Springs Hospital, you never knew what to expect. In the year I started there, the emergency department saw 43,033 patients, in a town that only had a population of 27,000. The hospital doesn't just service the town, it also takes patients from the surrounding remote Indigenous communities, some of which are hundreds of kilometres away.

I started my placement in the surgical ward and then moved on to the emergency department and maternity ward. In the ED I met a patient who came in with a urinary tract infection. It was a serious one and she must have been in a lot of discomfort, but it was easily treatable with intravenous antibiotics. While we sorted that out, the patient's relative who was with her asked if we could do anything about the patient's arm. 'What's wrong with your arm?' I asked her.

The patient said nothing, but her relative grabbed the arm in question and dropped it, so it swung around and flopped down at an obscure angle. It moved in a way that defied physics. An arm shouldn't be able to bend that way. It turned out that the patient's humerus had been broken four years earlier. She didn't seek treatment at the time because she lived on an outstation, hundreds of kilometres away from the nearest hospital. As such, the bone healed on an awkward angle that allowed her arm to swing in the most unnatural way. The movement was so confronting that when I called in the doctor (who had just started working at the hospital) to take a look, I could see the colour drain from her face. For a second, I thought the doctor might faint and I prepared to have two patients in front of me. The patient, meanwhile, remained unbothered. I didn't know whether that was because the injury no longer hurt her or if she had simply become used to the pain and accepted it. The doctor offered the patient the option of surgery to correct the break, but she decided to leave it as it was.

* * *

In Alice Springs there's the Camel Cup, the Finke Desert Race, the Beanie Festival and the Larapinta Trail. It's also known as the lesbian capital of Australia. I'm lucky to know and be friends with a number of people from the queer community but I've always thought of myself as straight. Until I moved to Alice Springs.

My housemate's name was Eve and we built a beautiful friendship. Eve was a social worker and I dropped off cups of coffee to her on my days off when she was working late. She returned the favour to me at the hospital. We went for a run together every afternoon. I wasn't a runner, but she taught me to be one. We bounced off each other, felt entirely comfortable next to each other, and missed each other when we were apart. We teased each other and shared a secret language of raised eyebrows. We were flirting, but I didn't know that, yet.

As all good love stories do, this one started with a bottle of Hennessy whiskey. After a house party, Eve woke up next to me in my bed. She froze. She didn't want to wake me up because she didn't want to see any signs of regret on my face. When I eventually woke up, I leaned over to give her a kiss on the cheek and then got up like it was no big deal. I think that deep down I always knew it was going to happen. I always knew Eve was going to claim a piece of my heart as her own.

It was all new to me. When I was looking into Eve's eyes, everything in the world felt right. I had fallen in love and was blissfully happy. But she was a she, a fact I was learning to come to terms with. When I was on my own, the doubts crept in.

'I don't associate with being gay – even to write it feels weird,' I wrote in my diary. 'I am with a girl – and she makes me happy – so the rest of the world views me as gay. I don't know how I feel about this. I do know the choices I make now will affect my future. I want to be a mum, and I could quite happily be with a man and make that happen. So why choose a girl when the world is so cruel? Why do I always have to take the hard road?'

As hard as it might be, Eve made the road feel worth the bumps and potholes. She was my safe space.

We were together eight months when I took a job as a remote area nurse (RAN). I didn't apply for the job. Rather, I did a three-day course in remote emergency care with a fantastic teacher who took a shine to me. Serendipitously, I was assigned to look after the teacher at the hospital when she was admitted as a patient some weeks later.

'When are you going to come out remote?' she asked me, as I was taking her blood pressure.

'I need a few more years of practice to even consider being a RAN. Those guys know everything. I'm just a baby nurse and midwife,' I said.

The teacher shook her head at me and insisted that I send her my résumé. I didn't waste time arguing as she was pretty stern. Two weeks later, I received a congratulatory email saying that I'd been accepted for a RAN position, on a pay grade two levels above what I was on. After extensive discussions with Eve and a deep look within, questioning whether I was really cut out for this – there was only one way to find out – I accepted.

Being a RAN, though, scared me shitless. It would be unlike anything I'd done before, and I felt totally out of my depth. As one of two RANs in the community, I would be responsible for the health and wellbeing of an entire town: 200 people. I'd be in charge of running the clinic, ordering supplies and keeping records. I'd also be the midwife for three expectant mothers. If something went wrong, help was a three-hour drive away. I would be on my own. And that terrified me.

I was seriously doubting myself and my abilities, and questioning the choice I'd made, but Eve came to the rescue. She talked me off the ledge.

'This is not about progressing your career. It's about progressing as a person. Being a nurse is what you do – not who you are. Being a nurse is the way you express your passion for fairness and justice, and your kindness and compassion for people,' she told me. Or, rather, she wrote it down in my diary, so I could read her words of support over and over again. I was going to need them.

The RAN program operates on three-month rotations. Nurses spend three months in a remote community, then three months back at Alice Springs Hospital, before heading out bush again. I told myself it was only three months, only twelve weeks, only ninety days.

* * *

In the flat vastness of the outback, a range erupts on the outskirts of the community. It took me an hour and forty minutes to climb to the top. There was no track, so I made my own through the spinifex and sparkly shards of mica that make the rocks shimmer in the sun. When I reached the peak, I had to catch my breath: 1) because it's a damn long way up, and 2) because the view is breathtaking.

'Shit, I really am in the middle of nowhere,' I thought to myself. There was nothing but red dirt and blue sky as far as the eye could see. It was spectacular. And it made me feel insignificant and tiny yet strong and brave to be standing there in such vastness.

It was my first week in the community and I was staying with my boss Karolien and her husband, Jason, until my own accommodation was ready.

The first place I went to when I arrived in town was the health clinic. Karolien was closing up for the day, so I got a quick tour before I started work in the morning. The set-up was very impressive. It was an old building, but there was a huge medical room, two offices, three treatment rooms, a waiting room, kitchen and laundry area, and showers and a toilet outside. Everything was clean and well organised.

My first day on the job felt like being back in kindergarten. Instead of a too-big uniform, I was wearing my scrubs. Instead of the alphabet, I was learning how to treat patients in a new clinic in a new town. I didn't know where anything was, had no idea how to use the computer system, and struggled to take anything in because it all felt so overwhelming. Karolien showed me the ropes and how to use the CARPA manual, and I was grateful to have a whole week with her to get my bearings. She was overdue for time off so was heading into town for the weekend, and I would then be left on my own. In my first shift, I treated six patients, ranging from scabies to antenatal checks, wound care to ear examinations and vaccinations.

I learned very quickly that being a RAN means you're so much more than a nurse. You're also a teacher; a counsellor listening to people's problems; a pharmacist; a stocktaker; a cleaner; a gardener; and a driver.

One woman had a severe mental illness that required her to take medication twice a day to keep her psychosis under control. Without it, she became a danger to herself and everyone around her. Her husband was a gentle, quiet man who was never far from his wife's side. It was the RAN's job to administer the medication, every day, twice a day. She hated taking the medication and hid the tablets everywhere she possibly could.

I used to drive to the Mount Ebenezer Roadhouse, an infamous pub on the Lasseter Highway. It was Friday night so I headed there for dinner. I took a risk and ordered the caesar salad, which was actually very good. It was a roadhouse miracle!

Sometimes after a call-out late at night, when I eventually crawled back into bed, I would feel the adrenaline coursing through my veins. I would be buzzing. I would force myself to lie still and slow down my heartbeat, but sleep evaded me anyway. It would often be 4 am when I finally closed my eyes, only to open them again a couple of hours later when my alarm went off.

* * *

Back at the clinic, the patients started coming in and they didn't stop. I organised my first medical evacuation for a non-urgent case. Sadly, it was for one of my pregnant patients who was bleeding and experiencing a miscarriage. We notified the Royal Flying Doctor Service (RFDS) and they planned to pick her up on their way back from another call-out from Yulara to Alice Springs. I squeezed her hand and wished her well. There was nothing I could say to make the situation okay – it was a devastating loss – so all I could offer was my sympathy and care.

The afternoon sped by in a blur. A young woman came in complaining of discomfort 'down there'. I took a urine sample and sent it off for a nucleic acid amplification test, crossing my fingers that it came back negative for any sexually transmitted diseases. I inspected a couple of boils, treated an allergic reaction in a six-year-old who was playing with a furry caterpillar and rubbed his eye, and dealt with some less 'urgent' cases. Some people really do seek treatment for the most ridiculous things. There was the bloke whose wound was itching (because it was healing). The teenager with a sore nose (because there was a pimple growing inside it). And the eighteen-month-old who kept falling over (because she was a toddler!). You had to laugh.

I saved up my work stories and told them to Eve when she came to visit me. These stories were easy to tell. They weren't all easy, though. I struggled to talk about the pain, loss and suffering I saw in my daily life as a nurse. Eve asked me how I coped with the vicarious trauma, and I told her, 'I don't know that I do. It's part of the job, you just have to deal with it.'

I have to be able to leave my job at work, I can't carry it with me everywhere I go. I'm not strong enough. No-one is.

Like any skill, the ability to cope with trauma is something you can learn, and you get better at it the more you do it. Interestingly, I can often feel more affected by other people's stories than mine. I could have a nurse colleague doing exactly the same job as me, and she could tell me the story and I'll say, 'That sounds so traumatic. That's really scary and really tough.' But then I would've been in the exact situation a week prior but to me that's not traumatic. It's not scary. It's just what you do, get on with things.

Over the years I have developed mechanisms to keep myself functioning at work. Swimming, running, journalling, reading. Wine too, although I'm trying to do that less!

* * *

Eve provided a happy distraction over the Anzac Day long weekend. We planned to meet halfway at a roadhouse and woke up early for the dawn service. The owner of the roadhouse ran the show. There were about ten of us who watched him lay a wreath on the fence. He was about to fire the gun in a salute when he stopped: 'Wrong bullets! I'll be right back.'

The service was followed by billy tea and 'gun fire breakfast' (coffee and rum). The roadhouse owner cooked bacon and eggs on the barbeque and Eve and I toasted our tea to the most unique dawn service either of us had been to. Only in the outback, eh.

* * *

One day I treated a very young patient with high blood pressure and protein in her urine, and she became critical. She had been feeling unwell and uncomfortable, and apparently had been putting on weight. She had been seeing a nutritionist about a weight-counselling program, but it hadn't seemed to help. She said she hadn't menstruated yet, but just to rule out pregnancy I did a pregnancy test. Two lines appeared. It was positive.

Her symptoms indicated pre-eclampsia, a multi-system disorder in pregnancy which can be fatal to mother and baby if not treated.

I continued with my assessment, measuring her fundal height as 36 centimetres, suggesting she was 36 weeks pregnant. I felt her belly and was relieved to find there were no signs that she was in labour, and then listened to the heartbeat, 136 beats per minute, suggesting a healthy infant was growing inside.

My job was to ensure the safety of everyone, including myself, so I prioritised the situation by first focusing on the patient. Since she had pre-eclampsia and needed urgent treatment, I contacted the RFDS and was put through to an obstetric consultant to make a plan. The RFDS would organise a transfer and the pile of mandatory reports I needed to fill out would have to wait.

The patient's blood pressure rose to 160/120, requiring urgent treatment for a potentially life-threatening condition. She was very unwell. It was at this point that I needed to ask her visiting family members to leave the room. I checked once more to see if she was starting to go into labour, and was again relieved to find that she was not. I gave her four massive needles, including two cannulas and two shots of magnesium straight into her thigh – which is incredibly painful. She didn't flinch.

The RFDS plane was an hour away. We had to go, the airstrip was an hour's drive away. We put the patient on a stretcher and loaded her into the back of the ambulance, which was a LandCruiser troopie. I grabbed the emergency obstetric kit and jumped in the back with her. Her mother was in the passenger seat next to Jason, Karolien's husband, who was driving us to the airstrip. We didn't put the sirens on; there was no-one around to hear them. Jason floored it. Somehow, we arrived at the airstrip before the RFDS plane, and I felt a familiar wave of relief when I saw it in the distance.

As the plane circled above us, the patient's mum grabbed my arms and whispered in my ear.

'Do you think it's a sign?' she asked me.

'A sign of what?' I said sympathetically.

'I had a miscarriage not long ago. Maybe this happened because there was already another one on the way?'

'That's a beautiful way to look at it,' I said, pulling her into a brief hug.

After the plane landed, the medics strapped the patient in and her mum took a seat on the plane before it lifted off in a great gust, leaving Jason and me standing there in the outback, covered in dust and still in shock.

The whole ordeal made my desire to be an RFDS nurse even stronger. So I reached out to them and followed up about the résumé I had sent them earlier in the year. The woman on the other end of the phone said she remembered seeing my résumé when it came in, and she told me I should soak up as much experience as I could, hinting at a possible casual role in the future. I did as I was told.

Working in these communities had fuelled my goal of joining the Royal Flying Doctor Service, and my dream of working with Médecins Sans Frontières was still boiling underneath.

* * *

The desert cold stings. It was the first day of my first winter here, and didn't I know it. My cheeks and fingers felt numb on my way to the clinic. The chill wormed its way into my body, and it took me all morning to warm up. I was rubbing my hands together, trying to get some feeling into them, when a patient arrived looking worse for wear.

It was another day, and another emergency evacuation. This one was entirely different to the last. The patient was eighty-nine years old and presented with generalised abdomen pain. It could have been any number of things: constipation, a urinary tract infection or appendicitis. Somehow, I managed to put a 24-gauge intravenous catheter into a tiny vein. It was a small win for me. The patient stayed stable on the drive to the airstrip. Another win. But when the RFDS medics arrived, we still didn't have a diagnosis, and after they flew away I didn't hear any more about the fate of the patient.

It was hard not to get attached. Working in such a small community and being so far away from anything else, you got to know people well and quickly. I became invested in their lives and health and families. Bonds were made, loads were shared, and respect was earned.

I was learning, too. I took notes from patients and the Indigenous healers in the community about bush medicine. A woman came into the clinic smelling of crushed leaves from the traditional medicine she'd been using to help heal a cut on her arm. Karolien taught me how to incorporate bush medicine in my treatments at the clinic using rubbing medicine purchased from the community. It was incredible knowledge to have and the experience was something I didn't take for granted. I didn't take any of it for granted.

Still, there were moments when the small town felt very small. In my quiet, big house, I sank into my thoughts and got tangled up in them. I wrote a list of all the downsides of working remotely:

1) I hate driving long distances.
2) I miss Eve.
3) It's lonely.
4) Although the experience is great, it is not ED, which is better recognised.
5) The responsibility is huge.
6) I really miss Eve.
7) There's so much to get done and never enough time.

I allowed myself to wallow for a moment, and then I did something about it. The timing couldn't have been better: I took a long weekend off work and drove straight to the train station in Alice Springs to meet Mardi and her friend Sue who were travelling on the Ghan train together. Yes, Sue, the very woman who told me to chase my dreams, and not to settle for being an air hostess when I could be the pilot. The train was late, so I only got three hours with Mardi and Sue during their stopover in Alice Springs. We saw the sights: Anzac Hill, the Telegraph Station, Honeymoon Gap and the Claypans at Ilparpa. It was a whirlwind tour and they loved every bit of it. I told them of my woes and passion and they gave me the talk I needed to hear before I waved them off at the train station for the last leg of their latest adventure and hoped I'd made them proud.

When I got back to work at the clinic I had an experience worthy of Mardi and Sue. I was called out to Yulara, the closest town to Uluru. Normally there's a population of 1000. At that time, there were 6000 people in town. Including the Dalai Lama! His Holiness had come to visit Uluru-Kata Tjuta National Park and meet the Traditional Owners. He made a speech to a crowd of 3000 people, and I was there to see it. I was in the centre of the country, listening to the Dalai Lama impart his wisdom – and I was getting paid for it. Pinch me.

My role was to provide support to the fatigued medical team, including Rod, the RAN who was first on-call. We both responded to a woman who was having difficulty breathing. Her voice was hoarse, so we cannulated her, gave her some medicine and monitored her closely. Then we treated a man who fell off a rock from a height of 20 metres. It had happened the day before, so he'd been lying out in the elements for twenty-four hours with three broken bones.

Rod was the definition of cool, calm and collected. He'd seen it all; been there, done that, and bought the t-shirt to prove it. Watching him work was a masterclass in nursing. I tried to absorb it all. I swear I learned more from watching other RANs work on the job than I did during my four years at university.

In my three months so far as a RAN, I liked to think that I'd become a better nurse – and person. Even on the hardest, loneliest, most intense days, I didn't take my experience as a RAN for granted. I only had two more weeks left and then I was meant to return to Alice Springs Hospital for another stint, before taking the rest of the year off to travel with Eve.

But before all of that, there were patients to see and paperwork to fill out.

I went out with a bang. The first day of my last week started with two emergency evacuations – one for suspected pelvic inflammatory disease, and the other for acute pulmonary oedema, a life-threatening condition involving fluid build-up in the lungs. We organised to meet an ambulance from Alice Springs Hospital halfway between here and there, as no RFDS planes were available. We handed the patients over to them on the side of the highway. It was all very high stress and major pressure.

I realised, though, that in some ways, I'd rather be there for the tough days. There was a guilt that came with dodging them. On a weekend when I was in Alice Springs, there was a car crash at Kings Canyon. Four Korean tourists were involved in the crash, three were in a critical condition and one was deceased. Karolien was the only RAN on-call in the area and one of the ambulances was broken, so there was also only one vehicle. Because of that, Karolien was told she wasn't allowed to leave the community to help at the crash site. The community couldn't be without a nurse or an emergency vehicle. It was protocol, but that didn't make sense. If I was there, one of us could have stayed and the other gone. I felt an extreme amount of guilt about this. Later I found out that the patients were able to get the help they needed from elsewhere and were transferred to hospital.

I tried not to think about that horrific accident on my way back to the clinic to start my shift that Monday. There was a line of patients waiting for me: a case of acute otitis media (a middle ear infection), a dog bite, gastro with abdominal pain, a new pregnancy needing follow-up care. I ended the day with the news of a missing 64-year-old woman at a nearby station. She'd been missing for twenty-four hours, so it wasn't looking good. I steeled myself to be called out to the worst, but the phone didn't ring.

It was a different story on my very last day of work: the phone didn't stop ringing. First, a mother called about her sick baby. Then there was a father who wanted me to tell his sons to go and visit him because he was in pain.

I celebrated the end of my contract with a roadhouse pub meal, where I heard on the local grapevine that the missing woman had been found. The police had set up a full-scale search with a dedicated grid and search party. They didn't have any luck. But a couple of local Indigenous trackers went out to look for her of their own accord and found her alive, albeit a little worse for wear.

There was a sign above the bar at the roadhouse saying 'Bull Bar', adorned with the skull of a bull. It was a fitting goodbye to a placement that I'd had to hold on tight for. As rodeos go, this might have been my first one in the outback, but it wouldn't be my last.

I'd done it. I'd survived my first posting as a RAN, and even though there were plenty of moments when I wanted to quit and run away, I didn't. I took the hard road, and made it to the other side. Though I got a few dings and flat tyres along the way. How's that for an outback analogy?

* * *

I had been meant to return to Alice Springs Hospital after I finished my three-month outback stint, but the bush called me back. I drove straight into a placement at a community a three-hour drive from Alice Springs.

On my first day at work, I was given a tour of the town by Jillian, my colleague and the local Aboriginal health practitioner (AHP). My accommodation was a very short commute to the office: twenty-one steps, to be exact. There were two RANs – my manager, Bryan, and me – and Jillian.

At the end of my first day, I offered to take on-call duty to give Bryan a break. When a call came in from a sixteen-year-old patient complaining of painful legs, things got real. It wasn't the case that jarred me, it was the reality that I was in a brand-new clinic, in a brand-new place and I didn't know where anything was or who anyone was. I needed to get some Panadeine Forte out of a locked medication cupboard, but I had no idea where the keys were to open it. I called Bryan, but he was out of reception on the road. I couldn't call Jillian because she didn't have a phone. Instead, I jumped in the work troopie and drove to her house to ask her where the key was before driving back to the clinic and finally opening the cupboard to get the medication. Thank god it wasn't anything urgent. It scared me to think how something so simple – opening a cupboard – could have been so disastrous. I spent the next morning opening every cupboard and learning every inch of the clinic. I felt calmer.

Which was lucky, because in my first week a ten-month-old baby arrived in respiratory distress with recurrent fever. It was evacuation time, but our airstrip was a daytime-only strip, and it was late in the afternoon. So with the RFDS plane unable to land, we reluctantly sent the patient home for the night after getting her temperature down with Panadol and stabilising her. In the morning, when the RFDS were on their way to transfer her to Alice Springs Hospital, she was tachycardic with increased difficulty breathing, with a temp of 38.8 degrees.

Organising evacuations had become second nature to me, and I still had a yearning to be on the other side. Both working with MSF and as an RFDS medic were still my priority dream jobs but I knew I needed more experience under my belt. That was why I was here.

I also started a university graduate certificate course in rural and remote healthcare to further my knowledge and bolster my résumé. In one of my assignments I was asked to name a health issue facing remote communities. I wrote about the inflated food prices and how challenging it was to afford to eat healthily and feed a family in a place where the local store charged $9 for some broccoli.

'What's your reference for this?' my tutor asked.

'My backyard,' I replied, explaining that I was currently working remotely, seeing the issues first-hand and listening to the residents' concerns in person. There are some lessons that can't be taught from an academic textbook, and can only come from lived experience.

* * *

A month into my stint I fell into a case of the bush blues. It was a predictable cycle for me: the high of taking on a new challenge and exploring new areas gave way to the isolation of the outback and the fear of being alone. I wrote an entry in my diary: 'I'm having one of those "what am I doing?" moments in my life. It's scary out bush – and I think it's changed me. I'm more reserved and introverted. I feel alone even when I have company. I don't want to be like this. And I don't know why I am? Seriously – in complete contradiction to the way I'm feeling – my life now is pretty great.'

I was right about that: I had a fulfilling job, lived in an incredible part of the world, had adventures on the horizon and was in love with an extraordinary woman. Although, the latter was one of the things weighing on my mind. I was thirty, and although I'd always wanted to have a family and be a mum, that hope felt further out of my reach because I was in a relationship with a woman. I know same-sex couples can have children, but it's not a straightforward process. Nothing about being with a woman had been straightforward for me. I had been nervous to tell my family about Eve, but in three short sentences, my grandma Mardi put me at ease.

'Oh I can't wait to meet her,' Mardi said. 'You know, many of my friends had relationships with women back in my day, but they weren't allowed to show it. I'm happy for you; if it feels right go for it, Prue.'

Eve is an amazing person, and she made me blissfully happy. I just wished I could be more comfortable in my own skin and being with her. First things first, though, and I needed to pull myself out of my negative headspace. So I went for a run (something Eve taught me how to appreciate).

It was a still afternoon. The sky was a mural of pink clouds that looked like floating puffs of fairy floss. The sight was almost too beautiful to be real. I was running through the back tracks of the community, surrounded by mountain ranges and passing by rock wallabies. When I stopped to catch my breath, I took a mental picture of the view. I never wanted to forget this moment or this place.

Back at the clinic, I saw a sight I would rather forget: a small dog with large puncture wounds. The poor thing had been attacked by a bigger dog, and some locals brought it to the clinic to be seen to. I'm not a vet, but I sutured the wounds as best I could and crossed my fingers. It was a hard realisation that my training and the resources we had could only go so far.

On a rostered day off, I met Eve at Glen Helen Gorge, just outside of Alice Springs, where the Finke River splices through the MacDonnell Ranges. It is an oasis in the outback, a waterhole in the desert, and for me a much-needed break to the outside world. In the Dreamtime of the Arrernte people, Glen Helen is known as Yapulpa (or Yapalpe). It is a sacred place and part of the Carpet Snake Dreaming. It is said that a rainbow serpent lived in the waterhole in the Dreamtime. Now, it's considered sacred because the serpent might still be lying there.

When Eve arrived, we braved the dormant serpent – and the icy cold water – and went for a dip together. Wow. It was fresh with a capital F. We warmed up with an afternoon G&T in the sunshine, before setting up camp at the Finke 2-Mile campground, just down the road.

Is there anything better than a campfire under the stars? Oh, and there was steak and veggies for dinner and a generous glass of red wine. It was exactly what I needed.

After our campfire dinner, Eve and I talked about our desire to travel together and, after a few reds and lots of laughs, we decided we would both resign from our jobs. Eve got on board with my plan to have no plan and just arrive and follow the wind. We decided on a one-way ticket to

Mexico and to then travel south. That was it, that was the plan. The possibilities were endless, just the way I like them.

My three-month RAN contract had come to an end so with only eight shifts to go, and an adventure planned, I was ready but worried about the clinic finding a replacement in time. I felt a pang of guilt about leaving, but I trusted that everything would work out. So much of working as a RAN is flying by the seat of your pants, so it seemed fitting that this was also how I was leaving the job. In the final hour of my final shift, I found out that a new nurse was starting straight away. Phew.

The time had come to leave the Red Centre for Mexico and beyond. So after a wave goodbye and a promise to return, Eve and I were off.

* * *

Somewhere in the Southern Ocean, Antarctica

'No-one tells you about all the pink penguin shit.'

– Me

It was a spur-of-the-moment decision. Eve and I were knee-deep in our epic adventure travelling through Central and

South America, when a fellow traveller mentioned it was the end of the Antarctic cruise season. We hightailed it down to the Argentinian town of Ushuaia – which is the southernmost city of South America – to see if we could get a last-minute deal on a ticket.

Sitting next to Eve in an Ushuaia travel agency, we watched a slideshow of photos from Antarctica which the travel agent had put together. By the second slide, Eve and I were sold. We looked at each other and had a silent conversation.

'Let's do it,' said her one-sided smile.

'Go on,' my subtle nod replied.

A few minutes – and AU$6355 – later, we had tickets for the adventure of a lifetime to the White Continent.

But before our voyage was set to start, we had a few weeks to fill in. Someone suggested going to Patagonia and doing the W trek of the Torres del Paine National Park. So with no sleep we were on a 5 am bus to Patagonia. After a backpackers' open information night in Puerto Natales, we soon found ourselves signed up for the 'solo hard core' option of the O trek, not the W. Which meant just a few more days out there walking around the mountain before meeting up with the W trekkers. We had never done an unassisted trek before and had to hire all our gear and try to come up with meals for the next eight days. We only had our ASICS trainers and stupidity to guide us. Then we were off. Through trials and tribulations and pure joy and laughter we made it the whole way around, unscathed and with some pretty phenomenal memories in the bank. This would turn out to be the birth of a passion of mine to tackle multi-day treks all around the world.

During the trek Eve and I reminisced about all our adventures so far, from celebrating our birthdays in Oaxaca in Mexico during the Day of the Dead festival, to hitching a ride with a donkey-drawn carriage with a drunk milkman in Nicaragua. Climbing Acatenango volcano in Guatemala, spending days at sea sailing through the idyllic San Blas islands in Panama. We learned survival skills in the forest in Colombia, and spent a few nights in hammocks in the Amazon jungle, acutely aware of the plate-sized spiders lingering nearby. Partied all day and night at the Rio de Janeiro Carnival. We dived in the Cenotes in Mexico, the Blue Hole in Belize and later went dry-suit diving with the enormous king crabs in Ushuaia. On Christmas Day we explored the deep ocean in a yellow submarine in Honduras. We stood in awe and kissed at the Devil's Throat at Iguazu Falls and got lost in the remote city of Iquitos in Peru, danced in the streets in Argentina, drank Malbec wine in Mendoza. The memories are endless; I could keep going. We had the time of our lives!

* * *

So there we were, sitting on the observation deck of the Ocean Diamond Quark Expeditions cruise ship heading south, all the way south. My jaw was in a permanent state of openness, as we crossed the dreaded Drake Passage. It's one of the most dangerous passages in the world and takes about forty-eight hours to cross. The currents at its latitude don't meet resistance from any landmass, so it has the reputation of being 'the most powerful convergence of seas'. The Drake lived up to its hype. The waves were bigger than the boat. I felt so small, like I could be swallowed up by the sea and no-one would notice. I had a distinct thought that I might die before we made it to Antarctica.

Finally out of the window, on the portside of the ship, through the thick fog and rain, we spotted our first iceberg. It was enormous. The next one was even bigger, and the next, and the next. It was like a giant game of eye spy, only more epic. I couldn't quite believe what I was seeing.

Spoiler alert: I made it to Antarctica without being swallowed by the sea.

On our first trip off the ship, we stepped onto the continent of Antarctica. Alongside the group of intrepid travellers on the cruise, we walked among the penguins, whose poo stained the snow pinkish red because of their krill/fish diet, and who took a liking to Eve's purple pants and came close to check them out. We stepped over whale bones and trudged our way through the snow to the top of a hill to marvel at the scenery that is beyond comprehension. Our Quark boat looked insignificant and LEGO-like in the distance. A traveller from Germany poured each of us a cheeky shot of vodka as a welcome to Antarctica. The hard liquor warmed my insides, but my fingers stayed numb. Before we got back on the ship, we scrubbed our boots. It made the experience all the more real. We were at the edge of the Earth, in the elements, on the purest continent.

A highlight of the trip was the aptly named 'Polar Plunge'. Unfortunately for me, I lost a bet with the crew the night before the Polar Plunge. I can't remember what we were betting about, but I lost. I was reminded of the punishment when I was standing on the gangway in my bikini and light harness around my waist.

'Yo, Prue, you lost a bet,' said one of the crewmembers, referring to my arrogance of the previous night when I'd declared I'd do the plunge naked.

A bet is a bet. I took my bikini top off, fortunately this was enough and when I looked back up at the boat, I saw a line of camera lenses pointed at me. I dived. Deep. I screamed until I hit the water and was submerged in total silence. The freezing cold stole my breath and even when I made it back to the surface, it felt nearly impossible to breathe. I never knew cold could feel like this. I struggled to get back to the boat. I did an awkward breaststroke (emphasis on the breasts) with a frog-leg kick and reached the ladder. Waiting at the top was Eve with a massive smile and a towel.

This trip was the definition of awe-inspiring. But as my mind was being blown, my heart was being broken. I was entirely to blame. I'd had a lot of time to think. Too much time. The doubts that had been in the back of my mind had grown louder. Eve and I had planned to do a stint in Canada after our travels, but I didn't have work lined up there, and I was worried about taking a step backward in my career. I knew I wanted to work in humanitarian aid – that had always been my goal – and I was scared I'd miss out on that opportunity if I went to Canada. I told Eve that I had my heart set on working for Médecins Sans Frontières, and I shared my concerns about Canada.

'Why can't you do it all?' was her reply.

'I'm happy to ruin my life, but I don't want to ruin yours.' In my mind you couldn't have it all, a wonderful relationship and a dream job that involves being away a lot. I was narrow-minded and decided to focus all my attention to humanitarian aid, leaving Eve behind to explore Canada on her own.

Eve had given me her all, but I was not able to do the same. It was a harsh truth – for her and me both. She deserved better. I wondered if I was self-sabotaging, but deep down I knew I needed to do the right thing by Eve and end things sooner rather than later.

Our love affair started in the hot red desert, and it ended soon after Antarctica. Ice cold.

CHAPTER THREE

The Top End

'No matter how hard you fight it, you fall and it's scary as hell. Except, there's an upside to freefalling ... It's the chance you give your friends to catch you.'

– Dr Meredith Grey, *Grey's Anatomy*

Having only worked in desert communities, landing in the tropical heat of the Top End is a shock to my system. The airport is a bitumen airstrip with a storage cage for luggage and a toilet block with a resident cane toad. It may be in the same territory, but the tropical north is like nowhere I've been before.

A friend had been working up there and suggested I go there and work too. 'You'll like it, it's a good place to heal and get back into work,' she said, aware of my recent break-up and adapting back to life at home. And she was right.

Having become acclimatised to the dry heat of the desert, I'm not used to sweating so much. I'm also not used to seeing palm trees, or any trees that aren't scrub or white gums. Walking down the palm-lined main street, the locals acknowledge me with a wave and a smile.

While I'm playing spot the difference ... The health clinic is enormous compared to the ones I've become used to. My first morning there, the staff gather for a morning tea. There are thirty-six people – including three doctors – in the room. I count. It's a change from being a two-nurse show; a welcome change.

While I was travelling overseas with Eve, a RAN named Gayle Woodford, fifty-six, was on-call alone in the community of Fregon, in the APY Lands of South Australia, when she responded to a medical call-out. She was doing her job when she was raped then bashed to death by a repeat violent offender. The crime made front-page news in Australia, and the outrage, grief and disbelief were felt around the world.

I was in Buenos Aires when the story reached me, and even though I was physically on the other side of the globe, mentally I was on-call in an outback community, just like I had been for most of the year before, just like Gayle Woodford was when she was killed. I couldn't help but think of all the call-outs I'd done on my own and all the times I'd been completely alone in the outback. There's a reason we never turned the troopie sirens on; no-one is out there to hear them.

The case was horrific, and it rocked the RAN community to its core. It forced the entire industry to take stock and carry out well-overdue risk assessments. More than 130,000 healthcare workers, including me, signed a petition calling for better provisions to be put in place to protect us. Subsequently Gayle's Law was introduced, requiring a second responder to accompany practitioners on out-of-hours calls in remote areas. As nurses, it's our ethical duty to help people who are hurt; but we shouldn't have to risk being hurt ourselves.

As much as I didn't want to be afraid to do my job because of the depraved revengeful actions of one man, I was relieved to get a RAN posting in a bigger town, with more support and back-up. This was a good place to take stock and reflect on the past year. I had friends there and even got back into running.

In my first shift, I was managing the emergency department. That sounds impressive, but it really just means I was running consults from the ED room, which had a total of two beds. My welcoming committee of patients were suffering from chest pains, the flu and ear infections. It was a busy day, and when I got home – to my big empty house a few blocks away from the clinic – I was itching to tell Eve all about it. Then I remembered ...

I bought myself a $9.50 block of Old Gold chocolate in self-pity, and let the tears flow. Why couldn't I have it all?

After my first week back at work following eight months off, the weekend couldn't come soon enough. Saturday was the biggest day of the year: the local AFL grand final. Both teams had spent the week making elaborate banners showing off their team spirit. The game was all passion and prowess, and I got so caught up in the atmosphere and people-watching that I missed the final score.

At the game, I met a local Traditional Owner named Max who invited me and a bunch of other clinic staff to go with him to visit his Country the next day. In the car on the way there, I was alarmed to see a small fire burning on the side of the road.

'Don't worry, they're fire drops,' Max said, explaining that little fires were lit from a helicopter above as fire management. Cultural Burning has been practised by Aboriginal people for thousands of years to enhance the health of the land and its people. First Nations fire management involves the lighting of 'cool' fires in targeted areas during the early dry season between March and July, to reduce fuel loads and create fire breaks. From the Airnorth plane that flies in and out of the airport, the land below looks like a patchwork quilt of burnt and unburnt country. I'd never seen or heard of fire drops before and I found it fascinating.

We drove for two hours on a sand track before pulling up at a tiny outstation, with a simple homestead, an airstrip and a school. Max's family were sitting on the veranda weaving baskets when we arrived, and they welcomed us with big smiles. They told us about how they catch bush tucker and I was impressed with their resourcefulness and skills. We got back in the car and drove for another hour to an even smaller outstation. This was Max and his family's actual home, but because there was no water supply, no-one lived there full time.

After a swim in the shallow pools of the nearby river, we set up a picnic for lunch, threw in a couple of fishing lines and kept an eye out for crocs. Max told us it's safe to swim in the shallows, but that we should avoid the deep swimming holes because that's where the crocs live. I could see why the crocs lived there; the cool water sparkled under the sun and called to us to jump in. I forced myself to ignore the call. I'd been told that crocs can hide in just 10 centimetres of water – so even puddles were potentially dangerous up here – and I believed it. There was a reason we didn't see any croc-bite victims in the ED in these parts. Crocs here don't miss. If they get you, you're gone.

Living here was like living in an outdoor adventure show. One weekend I was learning about fire drops with a Traditional Owner, and the next I was on a boat with my new teacher friend and her family, catching queen fish in the ocean and collecting fresh oysters from the rocks on the shore of a remote island where our footprints were the only ones in the sand. We had asked permission from the Traditional Owners to step onto the island, and we set up a small campfire to cook the fish. With bush plates (made from dried grass) on the sand and a wedge of lime each, we picked pieces of meat from the freshly cooked fish and dropped it straight into our mouths like hungry pelicans. As the ocean tide came in, it washed the fire away.

My adventures were paused temporarily by patients. I was on-call from 8 pm to 8 am on Sunday night, and the phone rang at 8.40 pm and it didn't stop. There was a teenager with a sprained ankle, a five-month-old baby with breathing issues and an elderly woman with exacerbated chronic obstructive pulmonary disease. I treated them all and they were all home by midnight. I made it home, too, only to be called out again at 1.30 am to a patient with chest pains. By the time I crawled into bed, my eyelids were as heavy as bricks. I made a mental note not to spend a day out on the boat in the sun before a night of being on-call – regardless of how fresh the oysters are.

* * *

I was still thinking about the fire drops and the mosaic of burnt and unburnt patches of land when something almost serendipitous happened. I met a fireman who worked in Arnhem Land. He had the sun-kissed skin of someone who works outside and the eyes of a man who's seen more than he should have in his time. His name was Mark and it was his job to light the little fires from the helicopter. Sparks flew (sorry, can't help myself).

The first time we spent a night together, Mark and I stayed up talking on the couch until 2 am. There was no touching or kissing, but it felt intimate. The next night we spent together, I was on-call. We indulged in a dinner of sashimi cut from Mark's catch of the day, but before the meal was over, I was called out to a patient; a man who felt cold. He'd taken an entire box of Panadol. He arrived at the clinic to meet me at 9.30 pm, and by 10.45 pm he was on an evacuation flight to Darwin. It all happened very quickly. I worked as fast as I could to get him the help he needed, but I didn't know if it would make any difference in the end. If the patient had 50 grams of Panadol in thirty hours, like he told me on the phone, he would likely die. It's a brutal way to go. The liver shuts down first, turning the eyes and skin yellow. Then the kidneys lose function, the brain swells and more organs painfully fail before death arrives.

When I got home after midnight, Mark was asleep on the couch. He had waited for me to finish dinner, so we ate our sashimi in silence. He went to bed first (in the spare room) and after an internal debate I avoided my desire to curl up next to him and retreated to my own bed. It took me a long time to fall asleep, thinking of the hot man in the next room.

When sleep finally came for me, it was immediately broken by a call. Then another twenty-one calls between 1 am and 7 am from a mental health patient who needed reassurance. A good thing I didn't go and snuggle.

In the morning, I got up to find Mark in the kitchen making coffee and breakfast. We still hadn't kissed or touched more than an 'accidental' arm brush, but there he was, shirtless and wearing a pair of shorts in the morning light of my kitchen. It felt familiar and foreign all at once. When Mark left to go fight a fire, I got ready to go to the clinic. We didn't kiss goodbye. I was starting to think there might not be a kiss. Even so, he'd been a welcome distraction and confidence boost; it was nice to have that feeling again, to mend a broken heart.

* * *

After I came home from South America, I was feeling lost and confused – as break-ups generally have you feeling. I'd ended my relationship with Eve because I had this strong desire to do humanitarian aid work. I didn't want our break-up to be in vain so it was time to find the courage and inspiration to follow through with my dreams.

I applied to MSF, got through all the stages and received a life-changing email congratulating me on my success. I had just been offered my dream job, a job that combined my love of travel with my love of nursing and midwifery. I was so elated. Yet close friends and family were concerned, saying, only half joking, 'Signing up to work on the frontline in a war-torn country is totally normal post-break-up behaviour, right?'

My MSF training was scheduled for a week in Sydney, so I took the week off and left the tropical Top End for the big smoke. I said goodbye to the cane toad in the toilet block at the airstrip on my way out, telling him I'd be back soon. On the flight to Darwin, I noticed how the burnt patches of land were now a vibrant green of regrowth.

The MSF crash-course in frontline medicine was held in a nondescript building in the inner-west suburb of Glebe. There were twenty-three of us in the training – all like-minded, ambitious and adventurous. Everyone had a different reason for wanting to join MSF, but we all shared the same ideal: wanting to be where the need is the greatest. In the humanitarian space, MSF has a reputation for being fearless; they go where no-one else will. Two people in the group had already been placed. A midwife was off to Sierra

Leone and a logistician was heading to South Sudan in a week. It was as exciting as it was terrifying. I knew this would be the hardest and most rewarding thing I would do.

But first there was the training. It was a week of huge days: 9 am to 6 pm. We were given lessons on how many sandbags deflect bazookas, avoiding being kidnapped and generally staying alive in conflict zones. We attended talks hosted by current and former MSF medics on coping with trauma and dealing with mental health issues. And, every night after training, we all headed out for a beer to get to know everyone. It was here I met Ben, a seasoned veteran who would become my confidant and good friend. There was a certain energy to the group, we were all high on adrenaline at the thought of what was to come and apprehensive about the same thing. We wouldn't truly know what we'd gotten ourselves into until we were in it. And then it would be too late.

After training I had a month left in the Top End. When I landed at the airport, I headed straight into the ED and it was like I'd never left; that my trip to Sydney and MSF training was all but a fever dream. I got on with my day, eagerly awaiting my placement email which could come any day, and dreaming of the possibilities. I treated two dog-bite patients.

One had superficial wounds, the other not so much. One patient had huge gashes out of his right calf. I did what I could and organised a transfer to Darwin for further treatment.

When I got a message from Mark asking if he could take me out the next night, my cheeks flushed. I felt like a giddy teenager with a crush. I shaved my legs in preparation, and prayed to God that the chicken I ate at lunch was okay ... Food poisoning would be just my luck.

Mark picked me up from work and took me straight to his boat. The water was choppy and there was a thunderstorm brewing on the horizon, but we persisted. Mark had come prepared; he'd packed drinks, dinner and mango for dessert. We were licking the mango juice from our fingers when the looming storm hit. The rain fell hard and fast. We were saturated by the time the storm passed, but we couldn't care less. Our wet clothes came off. Then it was on.

We spent the night alternating between fishing and having sex, both acts stirring something primal in me. I knew I'd have bruises in the morning. At least I could genuinely say I got them out on the boat.

As we trawled around the island, the sea was glowing. There was phosphorescence in the water, lighting it up like glow-in-the-dark stickers. I was in awe.

In the morning when I stepped off Mark's boat, I went straight up the dock to the clinic to start work, trying to act normal. I felt everyone knew my secret. I managed to get home during my lunch break and had a much-needed shower.

The Top End had been a healing experience – a chance for time and space to reflect. It was exactly what I needed post epic travel, break-up, dream job and readjustment. I somehow had clarity that I was on the right path, even if I had no idea where that path was heading.

* * *

The email I have been eagerly awaiting comes. The email subject reads: TAJIKISTAN – KULOB – PAEDIATRIC HIV PROJECT – 12 MONTHS

I'm going to Tajikistan. Things just got real. I have several thoughts in quick succession. I'm sad I'm not going to Africa. I'm pleased it's somewhere new. I'm worried how my parents and grandparents will take the news. And I'm overwhelmed at the thought of working with kids. Sick kids. Dying kids.

Among all the mixed emotions, one thought looms large: Where the hell is Tajikistan?

CHAPTER FOUR

Kulob, Tajikistan

'She has tripped and she has fallen but she has also jumped and she has flown.'

– A diary entry

Can you believe it? I'm working for Médecins Sans Frontières. This moment has been eight years in the making. Ever since I saw that photo of MSF nurses working in Africa while I was at university in Bathurst, through all my stints as a remote area nurse in the outback, across all my travels from Saudi to Africa and South America to the literal end of the Earth, Antarctica, this was the dream. Don't wake me.

Jerkala Hospital is a shock. The old Soviet building has missing panels on the roof and an uneven cement floor. The building is freezing cold. It looks like it is – or should be – abandoned. And yet, it's the site of the area's main health clinic. I'm here – as a part of my mission in Tajikistan – to teach a lesson on safe needle disposal to the hospital's senior staff. When the doctors enter the training room, they're wearing the kind of fleece nightgowns your grandma puts on over her pyjamas in winter. They've paired the pink and green nightgowns with socks and thongs. These are surgeons – highly trained and ranked professionals – and yet they don't have proper uniforms to keep them safe or warm. I am a long way from home.

I can't believe what I'm seeing, in the same way I can't quite believe that I'm here; working in a country that I didn't know existed seven weeks ago.

I've been in Tajikistan for a few weeks and this is what I've learned so far ... Tajikistan is a country with a relatively low level of HIV prevalence, but one of the key problems is that the society does not have much understanding of the disease. MSF's work focuses on supporting children with HIV/AIDS and their families. Our work is as much about testing, diagnosis and treatment, as it is about raising awareness and sharing education about the virus, providing counselling to help people adhere to treatment, and screening for opportunistic infections. We're also working towards countrywide changes in HIV programming and infection control measures. HIV is so preventable – by having appropriate education on needle use and disposal, sterilisation of surgical equipment and checking of transfused blood products.

In Tajikistan, there's stigma attached to HIV-positive people, who often have to hide their status to keep their jobs and avoid mistreatment from neighbours and even family members. Talking about HIV is taboo. As such, our work is desperately necessary, but also quite difficult.

We are in the process of providing appropriate needle disposal bins and implementing a waste-management program within the area's hospitals. A huge undertaking and more of a developmental-type MSF project, not my expected emergency project. But very important all the same. We start by trying to teach a group of nurses and doctors about needle disposal in a freezing cold hospital where they don't have access to enclosed work shoes, let alone safe needle disposal bins yet.

* * *

Before Tajikistan, I spent a week with MSF training, eating and drinking in Bonn, Germany, with thirty-seven other first-time MSF employees from Canada, the Central African Republic, Uganda, Pakistan, Myanmar, America and all over Europe. One of my roommates had travelled twenty minutes to get there; we laughed when I said I'd travelled over twenty hours to get there. We were a motley crew of nurses, doctors, midwives, logisticians, epidemiologists, project managers, and water and sanitation officers. In between the usual management workshops, safety and security modules and stress prevention lectures, the trainers put us to the test. I won't give anything away for those who have joined MSF Amsterdam and are on the way to Bonn for training, but you're in for a treat. Remember to dress warmly and take a head torch. That's all I am saying as the unknown is what makes this training so unique and memorable.

During that training week we learned so much and most importantly formed some solid friendships. I was so grateful for this. As I found when on assignment, my friends back home had difficulty understanding me. It was those first missioners in that room who I found myself leaning on, and I felt understood.

* * *

During a stopover in Istanbul waiting to board my flight to Tajikistan's capital, Dushanbe, I bought myself a G&T at the airport bar and got talking to a traveller from New York. I introduced myself as an international humanitarian aid worker. It sounded foreign and weird coming off my tongue, but I sure liked the sound of that. The New Yorker bought me a shot of tequila on my way to the gate. It didn't do much to calm my nerves. *Here I go*, I thought. From my window seat, I could see the snow-capped mountains in the light night sky.

At Dushanbe Airport, there was a line of vehicles and a group of drivers waiting at the exit doors, yelling out, 'Taxi, taxi, taxi.' Someone pushed through the crowd.

'Prudence? My name is Farid, I'm your MSF driver,' he said, showing me his ID and leading me to a four-wheel drive with the MSF logo on the side. It all felt very official and real. This was actually happening. I was in Tajikistan, and it was freezing.

* * *

It was 5 am local time and people were out sweeping the streets, which were dusted with snow. I was taken to a guesthouse where I met the medical coordinator of my project, Jai. After a brief rest I went off to the hospital for an HIV test and a quick introduction to people at the Dushanbe office. Then I was ushered into the back of a troopie for the four-hour drive to Kulob, where I would be based. I spotted goats, donkeys, cement houses, endless snow-capped mountains and women dressed in colourful clothes before I surrendered to my tiredness and closed my eyes.

When I opened them again, we'd reached our destination. The city of Kulob is quaint for a place that has a population of 100,000. It's surrounded by foggy mountains and full of decorative window trims and sporadic mosaic walls. You can feel the influence of its Soviet past. Most people speak Tajik and Russian. It's a beautiful place.

My house had a sauna and a courtyard with a seasonal pool and decorative fountain. My room was separate from the main house and involved a very crisp winter walk across the courtyard to the bathroom. This luxury wasn't what I was expecting when I signed up for MSF, but I was told this wasn't the norm by my five housemates, Gerrit from the Netherlands, Ahmed from Jordan, Sonia from America, Endashaw and Patrick from Ethiopia, and Lisa from Italy, whom I was replacing. 'Enjoy the luxury while you can,' Gerrit said. 'Your next mission won't be like this one.'

The office was a large compound with a logistics department, meeting rooms, kitchen, tearoom, dining room and a garden. I met the team, which was made up of six international staff (including me) and thirty-one national staff, many of whom had the most glorious names. There was a midwife on my team named Ozodamo, a lab tech named Tolibshoh, a training officer named Rahimjon and an infection control coordinator named Khursheda. The people were so welcoming and kind. I was greeted with warm hugs and the women just kept trying to feed me. I was overwhelmed by the kindness and the job and appreciated the fact that everyone was patient and understanding, giving me time to learn and settle in.

After the obligatory tour, introductions and a particularly intense two-hour meeting with my manager Jai, lunch was served, a local dish called *osh* consisting of 6 kilograms of rice, 4 kilograms of grated carrot cooked in 6 kilograms of animal fat and topped with 2 kilograms of meat. As you would expect, it was delicious, and was served every Friday.

Even though this wasn't a fast-paced emergency assignment, there was a certain urgency to it. I was introduced to people as a specialised HIV paediatric nurse/midwife with extensive experience in coordination and infectious disease. All of which I felt were deviations from the truth. My list of responsibilities immediately grew; I was liaising with the Ministry of Health, presenting at conferences, writing the monthly medical report and training teams. There was a training of trainers approach where I would train local staff with the help of translators to enable them to organise training sessions at HIV wards, maternity houses, hospitals and blood banks. We taught basic hand hygiene, personal protective equipment usage, proper needle use and disposal and waste management; we also raised awareness about the prevention and treatment of HIV. To do this, however, we needed more translators and one of my first tasks was to hire some.

When I asked Farzin, a 55-year-old Tajik man, why he wanted this job, he answered with tears in his eyes. 'A man at home bored is a very sad man,' he said. Naturally, I hired him. Not just for his tearful answer – I swear! – he also had the highest scores in his application test. Then I hired the beaming and genuine 22-year-old Suhrob, who quickly became my friend and direct line of contact for pretty much everything.

One month had already passed, and what a month it was, physically, emotionally and spiritually. I had become accustomed to the warm gold-toothed smiles and the warm greetings of right hand over heart with a nod, and I started responding in the same way.

I wasn't experiencing culture shock, so much as culture awe. I attended a match of the traditional sport known as *buzkashi*. Horse-mounted players attempted to place a headless goat into a goal. There were limited rules and no boundaries. The result was pure chaos and entertainment.

I love cooking, and enjoyed preparing meals for the team. These were quite elaborate – roasts and stews and whatever I could source from the market that day. One Sunday at the market I was intrigued and at a loss as to what some of the weird and wonderful looking vegetables (or was it fruit?) were. I had no idea, so I bought a few of everything and spent the entire Sunday in the kitchen with music on, frying, boiling, roasting, trying it raw. It was an entertaining day as I still have no idea what I was doing, but it would probably be the equivalent of boiling a pineapple, eating potato raw and frying a passionfruit. To say the least, my team was underwhelmed at the lack of edible food that night, so we quickly all jumped in a troopie to go to our favourite restaurant at a petrol station, which served my favourite borscht, a beetroot soup/stew. Delicious.

I was blown away by the Tajik people's hospitality and kindness to neighbours. We were all invited to people's homes for celebrations, whether a birth or a death, or just because. These occasions were celebrated with elaborate feasts, where we all sat on cushions on the floor, in a room with no furniture, with the food spread elaborately down the middle of everybody.

I attended a celebration of the birth of our MSF driver's baby daughter – where a massive spread of food was served for family, friends, neighbours and colleagues. During these events the men and women are separated, as is their culture. However, I seemed to be the exception, with the translators and most of my colleagues being male I was encouraged to join both the men's and women's areas during these events. Quite a privilege. The baby was passed around and we all told her how adorable she was and squeezed her chubby cheeks.

I also attended a celebration of death: the death of an MSF cashier's mother. Her beautifully presented body was laid in the centre of a room surrounded by many women supporting one another in quiet prayer. It is custom for the

family of the deceased to provide food on three occasions –
three days, forty days and a year after the death. I naturally
gravitated to the room where the women were congregating
to pay my respects, and later outside got talking to an eight-
year-old girl and her fifteen-year-old sister, who taught me
how to count to ten in Tajik. On both occasions, I left with a
full stomach and a full heart.

Then, I attended a celebration of love. The wedding of
Sobina, twenty-one, and Sady, twenty-three, was an eleven-
hour affair, with traditional dancing, customs, and copious
amounts of food. Sobina, the bride, wore a huge dress for
her big day. At twenty-one years old, that day she would get
married, leave her childhood home, move into the groom's
family home and consummate her marriage. She confessed
to me that she was nervous, and blushed when I asked her
about the car ride from the ceremony to the reception, which
was the first time she'd been alone with the groom.

'He kissed me,' she said through giggles.

'On the lips?'

'No! On the cheek.'

Her innocence was remarkable. We drank sugar water in
honour of the bride and groom to wish them a sweet life.
Cheers!

* * *

I was thinking of what my own sweet life might look like when I got a message from James. He couldn't sleep so he called me, and we spoke for an hour and a half. We chatted about everything and nothing. James reminded me what an incredible adventure I was on and I agreed with him. When we eventually hung up, I wrote an entry in my diary: 'I am so going to marry that man one day. Well, I seriously would like to marry him. He is the love of my life. We just need to trust our paths will cross again.'

James was my safety net. When I felt alone and adrift in the world, I still found solace in the fact that he existed. The image I had of him in my mind was a fantasy, but it was something to cling on to. He was living his own dreams but we stayed in contact throughout the years and, although we both had been in and out of love, I still felt a familiarity and deep respect for him.

* * *

I quickly developed an adoration for Tajikistan – the people, the culture, the food and the landscape. And I became very familiar with the unique quirks of the place. For example, the locals don't drink cold water because they think it will make them sick. But the room-temperature water there is naturally cold because it's freezing! The locals eat pomegranates like we Aussies eat apples and oranges: regularly. I would buy 5 kilograms of pomegranates at a time at the markets for 100 somoni (approx. AU$16), and I ate them every day I was there. The ceremony of pulling out the seeds and eating a pomegranate became very therapeutic.

Kulob is a city, but really, it's a small town. Everyone knows everyone; the corner store worker goes to school with the MSF driver who is best friends with the teacher's mother. There's a wonderful sense of community, respect and love, and I felt special being there and sharing in it.

There are four proper seasons in Tajikistan: the white, the green, the yellow and the brown. I arrived during winter and spent the months in awe of the white landscape, the magnificent views and the snow squelching underfoot as you try to keep your balance. On sunny weekend days I would drag the expats out to go picnicking in the snow a short drive away up in the hills.

One day I convinced Gerrit to join me on a run. He took a bike and we headed out for the afternoon for a 16-kilometre walk/run/ride. Not long into it we met Faiziddin, a young bloke also on a bike. He joined us and practised his very impressive English. Even to the point of asking me why I lived there and didn't speak the language. To him that was very stupid; I had to agree, my choice to learn Russian seemed really dumb when I lived in a Tajik-speaking town.

The more I fell in love with Tajikistan, the more I wanted to travel around the area. I ended up in Kyrgyzstan for a conference. I met up with some fellow MSF workers based in Bishkek and we hired a car and travelled around Issyk-Kul, the world's second largest saline lake after the Caspian Sea. We went to the largest animal market in the world and found ourselves on horseback riding in the snow-covered mountains admiring the views.

We spent a day skiing at Karakol. This place was so unbelievable that photos don't do it justice. For a huge $35 we got a ski lift pass and ski hire. The Europeans headed straight down the slopes, but I was an amateur, so one of the Swiss women, Justine, stuck with me, laughing at me the whole day while I fell over, spending most of the time on my arse running into trees and getting spectacularly lost.

During that trip we stumbled upon the town of Cholpon-Ata, where there was a huge street party celebrating Navruz.

There were nine yurts decorated with the symbols of the nine different tribal groups, each with different dress, dance, food and customs. We stuck our heads into the small opening of the yurt and before we knew it we were surrounded with people proudly feeding us an array of their local dishes. I ate horse, horse innards soup, horse stomach and horse some-other-body-part. (You learn to stop asking questions.) Not forgetting the vodka shots – my gag reflexes were certainly put to the test that day. We danced, we laughed and were laughed at when trying to learn the local dance. It was magnificent.

* * *

The love I felt for Tajikistan unfortunately didn't extend to my job. I had many discussions with Ben from my Sydney MSF training days, who had been in similar situations and was an absolute godsend when it came to talking things through. The reality of my role was far from what I had hoped it would be. When I applied to join MSF, I did so wanting to be in the thick of things, working with the patients who need the most help and collapsing to sleep at night in total exhaustion. Instead, I was sitting behind a desk for eight hours a day, five days a week. I'd avoided desk jobs for ten years, and now in the one job where I thought there would be zero chance of sitting behind a desk all day, there I was doing just that – I just had to go to *Tajikistan* to do it. In six weeks, I'd laid eyes on one patient, whom I wasn't allowed to assess. I bit my tongue.

In my bedroom late that night, I put on an episode of *Grey's Anatomy*, and had a stern chat to myself. Could I really do this for an entire year? I loved the place absolutely; I adored the people, the food, the scenery. But the job satisfaction was non-existent. I remembered working in the disability home in England and how it took three months to settle into that. I told myself to wait three months, then decide.

To feed my need to interact with people, on Saturday mornings Gerrit and I would head down to the English school and teach the students English. This is where we first met Sadi, who organised the teaching. In cold cement rooms painted a bright yellow with simple furniture and not a spare seat in sight, we would stand up the front and teach. Gerrit taught with slideshows and pictures of his home country, the Netherlands. I took a more practical approach and taught basic anatomy and basic first aid, including how to stop a wound from bleeding, how to keep it clean and the recovery position. In a break someone would inevitably start a snow fight. So much laughter and fun with the kids.

I was an acute nurse, not a chronic one. I worked on the frontline, not in the office. I thrived under pressure, not paperwork. The project in Kulob was a long-term change, so it would take years to recognise any change and see the impact of the work. It became quite obvious to me and my manager that I was not suited for such a project. I'm not a quitter, but I wasn't made for a job where I counted down the hours each day, either. Every hour that I counted, I could feel my patient care skills slipping by. Something had to give.

In the end, the project leader at MSF made the call for me. He told me that I was fully capable of doing the job, but his aim was to maintain first-time missioners. He said he was concerned that if I stayed in Tajikistan in this mismatched role, I would burn out and it would be the only MSF assignment I did. That wasn't what MSF wanted, or what I wanted. A decision was made: MSF would find a replacement for me, I would stay to hand over to them, and then I would apply for my next assignment, something more emergency-centred. I was relieved and devastated at the same time. I felt like a failure.

After this discussion I found myself cherishing every moment because I had no idea of how long I had left. I hoped for a few more weeks. I was acutely aware that the next place I went would be challenging in all sorts of new ways. I hoped I had what it takes. I knew that when sleeping in a hut fighting off mosquitos with no sleep I would be dreaming about Kulob and questioning why I'd left. This assignment had knocked my confidence and although I'd been reassured by all my bosses that it wasn't a failure, just a mismatch, and these things happened, it still wounded my soul.

The day I told the staff I was leaving was an emotional one. The nurse, Lola, and the midwife, Ozodamo, came and gave me massive tearful hugs. They were shocked by the news, but they understood my reasons.

'It's a very sad day,' said our MSF driver, a gentle giant of a man.

'We don't want to see you go, we respect you so much,' said another.

And my favourite response: 'I want to punch you in the face,' said Suhrob, with a smirk. He said it with love!

In Tajikistan International Women's Day is an official public holiday. As it should be everywhere. Women are congratulated and given roses for being the amazing creatures we are and for our ability to grow human life. I had woken up to a stream of messages, including this one from someone I met briefly at Sobina's wedding.

'Good morning, Miss Prudence. I am Izat, do you remember from the wedding day? How are you? How is everything? I hope you are doing good. Congratulations ... Happy Mother's Day. Dear Prudence, wish you all the best, success and happiness in your whole life. We appreciate you for everything and I hope you great feeling and the best experience being with Tajik nation hopefully on your mission in Tajikistan. With great respect and best regards, Izatullo.' How could you not love this place?

It is custom to spend part of the day visiting the elderly or the sick, so I tagged along with a local colleague to her frail aunt's house, where four generations of women came together. We sat on the floor and ate glorious homemade food served on huge wooden dishes. *Qurutob* – a heavy bread, oil and cheese dish with onions and herbs – was the centrepiece, all shared and eaten with the hands. It was a remarkable experience, and a humbling one.

I wondered whether I was mad for leaving such a beautiful community, a safe assignment and an unsatisfying job for something that could well be the complete opposite. I didn't have time for doubts, though. Four months after arriving in Tajikistan, an email landed in my inbox. The subject line read: ETHIOPIA – PUGNIDO/TIERKIDI – MIDWIFE ACTIVITY MANAGER – 9 MONTHS

CHAPTER FIVE

Pugnido, Ethiopia

'It's not quite the end of the world, but you can
see it from there.'

– Imtaiz, human resources officer, MSF briefing

I'm following a trail of blood into the Pugnido medical centre. Dark red pools lead me to the delivery room in the maternity ward. It's my first Sunday – my day off – and I had been eating breakfast with Will, a fellow MSF nurse, when he answered a call requesting urgent assistance at the hospital. I go with him and that's where we find the blood. So much blood. Too much blood.

In the delivery room, we rush to a patient who has presented with an antenatal bleed. She is soaked in the blood that led us here. The midwives have inserted two IV cannulas and are running fluid and put in a catheter – they've also given her paracetamol – but the woman desperately needs a blood transfusion and surgery. This medical centre isn't equipped for that, so she needs to be sent to the hospital in Gambella, a four-hour drive away on a pothole-ravaged dirt road.

The patient will be transported in a shelled-out troopie that's been forged into a makeshift ambulance with a stretcher in the back. That's it. There are no sheets or pillows. A rubber glove is used to tie the fluids bag to the ceiling. A midwife will join her for the trip. We hope the mother can survive with this much blood loss. We hope and we pray, because there's only so much we can do.

Before the 'ambulance' can urgently set off, we need to get permission from the Administration for Refugees and Returnee Affairs (ARRA). You see, the patient is a refugee, and she cannot travel without a permit. Life, death, permits. This is Pugnido.

The town is situated in Western Ethiopia close to the South Sudan border and is home to a refugee camp housing 50,000-plus South Sudanese people who've fled conflict in their homeland. The town has a medical centre with a paediatric and medical ward, an emergency room, an ICU (which just means there's access to oxygen), and a maternity ward with a delivery room and antenatal and postnatal beds (where I would be spending most of my time). The clinic provides care to the whole population in the area; it serves both the host and refugee population, regardless of their geographical origin, tribe, family or religious background.

There's also a health post in the refugee camp, known as Pugnido 1, where hundreds of patients are seen each month and referred on to the hospital if necessary. More serious cases are referred to the hospital in Gambella, where my patient is heading on that bumpy dirt road. This is the road I followed to get to Pugnido two days ago: in a troopie with eight other people and all our luggage. I pray that my patient's trip is smoother and faster than our four-hour trip.

I arrived in Pugnido with a sore bum, a serious case of jetlag, and a welcome-to-Africa bout of diarrhoea. It was a relief to find I had my own ensuite in the MSF compound I'd be calling home. There were eight bedrooms in the big cement building, a traditional *tukul* (round home) with couches and a TV, and a communal kitchen and dining area. It was a welcoming and pleasant space. A cook came every day except for Sunday and made rice, beans, meat stews and bread for us. A milkman delivered one litre of fresh cow's milk in a Coke bottle every other day, which we had to boil before we could drink it. My room had a single bed with a mosquito net and some simple plastic furniture. There was no internet and the power was patchy. The electricity generator shut down at 4 am every morning with a final 'click click' of the portable fan beside my bed. The stillness set in and the sweat dripped off my forehead.

My housemates were transient, coming and going from all over. Emma, the new project coordinator from Scotland, was taking over from Will from the UK. Will had been there for eleven months and was the current backbone of the medical centre where we all worked. Will had kind of been a one-man show, he was the nurse, the medical team leader and the project coordinator as staffing had been an issue. For the past six months, the hospital had been without a midwife, so he'd been filling that gap even though he didn't have midwifery training.

It was incredible to watch him work; the way he interacted with the staff in a number of languages, how he knew where everything was, and the skill he had to solve any problem, answer any question and generally get the job done. His work was second nature to him; a job that would take one of us newbies an hour, took him minutes. Will was the link between the national staff and the hierarchy above. I stuck close to him and hoped some of his knowledge would rub off on me. He only had two weeks left of his placement in Pugnido, so I knew I needed to make the most of that time.

I was in good company there: the international staff all shared a similar attitude and sense of adventure. The camaraderie was what I had expected from MSF. I was running the maternity ward and had been tasked with the job of upskilling all the MSF and the Bureau of Health (BOH) midwives in preparation for the bureau to take over from MSF. I had four months. I didn't know that yet, though; the transition was spoken about as something in the distant future. It was happening, but we didn't know when – or how. It was my job to be ready.

On Sundays in Pugnido we had to fend for ourselves meals-wise, so I was on a mission to make mashed potato. Who doesn't love a nice, creamy mashed potato? And all you need is potatoes; yes, we had plenty. We had some milk, and then we needed butter; hmmm, no butter. Where does one source butter from, at the end of the world in Pugnido? You couldn't buy it, so perhaps we could get someone to churn it for us, but who and how? The desire for mashed potato went unsatisfied. But the team didn't forget. I had planted a craving. Our obsession with creamy, delicious mashed potato grew and grew. Our logistics guy, bless his soul, had a planned meeting in Gambella, so off he went, secretly taking an esky we used for keeping medications cold. To our absolute delight he miraculously found and brought back butter. Four blocks of it in fact. So, with our Sunday dinner plans prepped, the week couldn't finish quickly enough. And yes, it did satisfy all cravings.

Pugnido itself is a lush green oasis, with nearby rivers, plenty of donkeys and goats, and people dressed in bright outfits. As MSF workers, we were lucky that our safety was not under threat here. We were not working in an active conflict zone, rather helping the people who had been displaced by conflict. Though, in my second week, I heard a man was killed by a lion 20 kilometres out of town. The story spread through the town like wildfire. I don't know if it was true or a tale made up to screw with the foreigners, like drop bears in the Australian bush. I wouldn't have been surprised either way. The reality was we were living in a national park in the wilds of Africa.

Still, we had the freedom to wander into the Agnuak village, pull up for a beer and order a meal of local food. The waitress at our local haunt was a vivacious twelve-year-old girl who served cold beers with the biggest smile. That's the thing about smiles, they're universal, they cross all language and cultural barriers.

Walking through the town there were sometimes cattle tied up in the main street. I asked what that was all about and learned it was tomorrow's food. They were to be slaughtered in the early morning, the meat shared between many vendors and then cooked and served to the people. *Shekla tibs* was my favourite.

Unsurprisingly working as a midwife in Ethiopia is entirely different to doing the same job back home. I still considered myself a baby midwife when I went over, I had dealt with many pregnancies in a place with help close by and a more definitive health service a flight away if I was out remote. However, in Ethiopia help was not close by and our definitive hospital was less than ideal. I could have been a midwife in Australia for forty years and would have never been prepared for working in Ethiopia. Multiple pregnancies, breech deliveries, STIs, sexual gender-based violence (SGBV), abortions, miscarriages, malaria causing preterm deliveries. The most heartbreaking part was feeling helpless with limited resources and knowing the women had little to no choice in reproducing.

So many women have the choice of contraception – to have an active sex life and not have the consequence of a baby – but we easily forget about the women who do not. The women for whom family planning is not an option, the women who have been raped. I had conversations with women in Ethiopia who did not want more children. They already had too many mouths to feed. I couldn't help them with this. We had condoms, that's it, and when offered to a woman, the response was: 'That's for the men to be educated on, that's for them, that's not for us.' Women's access to contraception was non-existent and the unplanned pregnancies could be life-threatening as there was limited access to basic care. They had no choice. Abortions were taboo and often unsafe. Mercifully, we did have the morning after pill for the SGBV victims so at least we could help those women who sought medical care within a certain strict timeframe, which was not always the case as it could sometimes take days before they reached us.

We also saw patients at the refugee camp health post. The camp was unlike anything I had imagined. It wasn't an overcrowded tent city brimming with desperation. It was an enormous green plain speckled with fenced mud huts, solid latrines, a preschool and school, and cows and goats. Women sat in the street wearing elaborate necklaces, watching their naked kids run around in glee.

The medical outpost was a shed with some cement floors. It was simple, but well set up. There were triage and consult rooms with malaria rapid diagnostic testing, a pharmacy dispensary, observation room and an antenatal room. There was a constant stream of people – how they managed such a scale of human need was impressive. With their limited facilities and resources I felt so privileged to join this hard-working team.

I was slowly learning Amharic, the most widely spoken Ethiopian language, and the one spoken by my team. 'Ameseginalehu' (ah-mess-seg-ah-nah-le-who) means 'thank you'. Yes, seven syllables, no shortening, no quick one-syllable version. I said it multiple times a day.

There were many other local languages. Our patients were mostly Agnuak from Ethiopia or Nuer refugees from South Sudan, and they all had their own languages. I learned pretty quickly not to confuse them after mistakenly greeting an Agnuak woman in Nuer. It did not go down well. Lesson learned.

I was the rookie here, but I was also the apparent boss. I walked the fine line between student and leader. I had so much to learn, and I made a conscious effort to sit back and watch how things were done. The national staff knew what they were doing, they'd been doing it for years and they were really good at it; the last thing they needed was another expat coming in and trying to assert their dominance with all guns blazing. I knew my place. Right now, my place was on the observation deck. I kept an eye out for things that worked and things that needed improvement. Instead of telling the team what to do, I sat down and listened to their suggestions on how to make their jobs easier.

The national staff had done their training here on the frontline, not in a well-resourced hospital in Australia. There's a big difference. In Australia, if a patient came in with serious blood loss, we'd do a blood transfusion. Here, that wasn't an option – we didn't have the equipment – so we needed to do what we could to stabilise the patient and organise transport to the hospital in Gambella. I knew how to do a blood transfusion, but I was still learning how to stabilise without equipment and how to sort transport to Gambella. I learned by watching. I listened to what the staff told me they needed, instead of what I might have thought they needed.

I was fully aware that the local team would teach me more than I would ever teach them.

However, after a few days, I realised I could help them

with something. After watching and learning it was evident neonatal resuscitation was not really practised and, after discussions with Emma and the team, it was decided it was an area that needed improvement. So, with this achievable goal in mind, I set out to teach all the staff basic neonatal resuscitation skills, following the MSF protocols. I held bi-weekly education sessions for the team, even the nurses and doctors from the hospital would come and join in. I learned to never let an opportunity pass to teach.

There were moments during my early shifts when I felt entirely out of my depth, but I didn't say that out loud. I didn't show my impostor syndrome on my face. I pushed it deep inside of me and got on with the job. The cover of the blank diary I'd brought with me was embossed with gold letters that said:

YOU

CAN

IF

YOU

THINK

YOU

CAN

I think I can, I think I can.

Back at the hospital, I was finishing up for the day. It was 5 pm and I was about to walk out the door when a mother ran into the clinic carrying a four-hour-old pre-term baby weighing 1.3 kilograms. Shit, I was immediately out of my depth, but with the help of the team we tried to figure out what we could and couldn't do.

We started giving the baby bag-mask ventilation. We didn't have any oxygen available to us. We did observations and somehow I managed to insert a cannula into the tiniest of veins and put in a nasal gastric tube. We started the baby on intravenous fluids, antibiotics and glucose. Then we set up 'kangaroo care' (where the naked baby is held to the mother's naked chest so it has direct skin-to-skin contact). It was all our facilities allowed us to do. It was late by the time the baby was somewhat stable, but I stayed on for a while longer, keeping a close eye on the fragile infant. The outlook wasn't good.

When I started work the next morning, I learned that he passed away at 1.15 am, and another baby with severe malaria died three hours later at 4.30 am. Two babies lost in a matter of hours. It was heartbreaking, but also completely normal here. Death is a day-to-day occurrence, especially with kids under five. Everyone seemed desensitised to it.

When the mothers left, there was no great ceremony, they just took their lifeless babies home.

* * *

On my thirty-second birthday I found myself with my whole hand and wrist inside a patient's vagina. The labouring woman had come in earlier in the morning with a breech presentation, it was a Sunday and I was called in to assist.

I took a poll of the three midwives on duty and between us we'd done about five or six breech deliveries. Of those, I'd done zero. Here we go …

The baby's body came out at 10.32 am, but their head was stuck. It was taking too long. We needed to get the baby out. An eerie sense of urgency filled the room. It must have drifted out the door and down the corridor, because soon a couple of doctors came in to assist. But the baby's head was stuck, a life-threatening situation. Sadly, minutes after we felt the heart rate slow to suddenly stop, we lost him. But we could still save the mother.

We could see a fluid-like sac on the baby's back. 'That's not normal,' I thought. We were all on overdrive, a room full of people trying to help, brainstorming how to get this lifeless baby fully out.

With maternal effort, external pressure and my hand inside her vagina trying to dislodge the head, it was clear something was terribly wrong. I kept pulling until my fingers started to cramp. This wasn't working. We began considering the options in this dangerous situation, and all of them were confronting. I felt for the mother with a lifeless baby remaining inside her.

A doctor suggested decapitation.

'No,' I said, 'because the head will still be stuck in the mother's womb.'

Another doctor said we could try capsizing the brain, which involves puncturing the baby's brain to empty the cranial contents and allow the soft bones to fold in on one another for the head to be passed through the birth canal. We didn't have the required equipment, but potentially we could make do with what we had.

The third option raised was a symphysiotomy, a surgical procedure in which the cartilage of the pubic symphysis is cut and released to widen the pelvis, allowing childbirth when there is a problem with the delivery like this. The procedure can have serious lasting effects and requires six weeks of bed rest to recover from, which wasn't possible for a mother of several children in a refugee camp.

'I don't want to put the mother through that.'

With the help of the MSF obstetric guidelines, we considered all the options. It was a surreal and difficult discussion to be having. I'd been there less than a month and I was talking about the potential of having to decapitate a baby. This was a dire situation, and the possible solutions were equally dire.

Meanwhile, we were still manoeuvring the mother to try to push the baby down. Eventually – incredibly – the baby budged. The head was delivered at 10.58 am, after the longest thirty minutes of my life. It immediately became apparent why the head had been stuck. The baby boy was deformed. His head was double the size it should be, his skull was enormous, and one eye was bulging out of the socket. The other eye was closed shut. Never to be opened.

It wasn't until later, when I was debriefing with a fellow midwife, Margot in Australia, about the case, that I found out the reason for the deformity. We worked out that the baby had spina bifida with hydrocephalus, which is often called 'water on the brain'. This extra fluid causes the brain to swell and become too large to deliver.

It was a confronting thing to see. Because of the spina bifida hydrocephalus, the baby was always going to be incompatible with life. No matter what we did, we wouldn't have been able to save him. But thankfully we were able to save his mother.

A delivery like this would never happen back home in Australia because of the scans, strict antenatal care and c-section option and the immense resources in our maternity wards. That's why I joined MSF: to help those without access to healthcare. This was the reality of that. It was a devastating, blood-soaked, brutal reality.

I took some solace in knowing the mother was physically okay. If she had delivered the baby at home without us, she may have died too. She was alive, but broken. I didn't know how she would emotionally recover from the trauma of the birth and the loss of her baby. Truth be told, I didn't know how I would, either.

I don't tell these stories for them to be read like trauma porn. I tell them because they need to be told, because this is the reality in so many parts of the world, and because I know how much I've learned from my experiences. There's power in knowledge – and hopefully compassion too.

I reminded myself that this trauma was not mine – I may have witnessed it and shared the experience, but it was not mine. My heart went out to the mother and family.

When I knocked off work, I headed to the local bar where earlier in the week I'd organised to meet my colleagues for a birthday drink. I was a mess and I hadn't had a chance to shower. The last thing I felt like doing was celebrating, but I forced myself to because my teammates wanted to make a fuss of my birthday. At the bar, they'd strung up balloons, toilet paper as streamers and leaves as decorations to mark the occasion. The tables were covered in lollies, and it felt like walking into a toddler's birthday party. I was grateful for the love – and the distraction – but I was shaking on the inside. I was in shock.

Physically, I was at a bar toasting my birthday, but mentally I was still in the delivery room with my hand inside my patient's vagina, tugging on her deformed baby. I tried to pull myself back to reality, but I couldn't. I hoped the horror didn't show on my face.

I tried to smile wide, and wider still when I was given a dress as a gift. It was thoughtful and beautiful. After dinner, fireworks and melting plastic candles were lit in my honour. Eventually I collapsed in bed, shattered in every sense of the word.

It was a memorable birthday for more reasons than one.

* * *

After Tajikistan and before Ethiopia, I spent five months at the family farm in Crookwell, soaking up the normalcy of home while waiting for my visa to be processed. Since I couldn't commit to any other work contracts I had the small blessing of time, time spent with my family at home, something I hadn't done since I was twelve. It was so fulfilling – I became part of the family again, arguing with my brother and helping out on the farm. During this time I also caught up with friends and went to some weddings and engagement parties, and I worked up the confidence to confront James. I needed to do this. As with any great romance, in my head we were going to be together, a belief I formed while I was living in Saudi, but he had no idea I felt this way. It was time to tell him. We'd known each other for more than a decade, and when we caught up at a mutual friend's party I summoned the confidence, with the help of a few drinks, to confront him.

'James, what are we doing?'

'I don't know,' he said.

'I'm putting all my cards on the table here,' I said, 'and it's up to you how you want to play them. You are the love of my life.'

Silence.

'When I see you, I see home,' I told him.

Silence.

'I see a future with you,' I continued.

More silence.

'Okay, we can talk about the weather now ...' I joked, trying to dig myself out of the sinkhole.

We spent an hour talking and avoiding the subject at hand. There was, however, no awkwardness. Strangely, I didn't feel rejected or left hanging (even though that's undoubtedly what I was), I only felt relieved and proud of myself for making myself so vulnerable. The ball was in his court. He knew how I felt; what more could I do? And if he decided he felt the same, he knew where I'd be: Ethiopia.

I did eventually get the all-clear on my visa and I was off.

* * *

A standard week in Pugnido goes a little something like this ...

Monday: I'm called into an emergency in the maternity ward at 10 pm. There are twenty sets of eyes staring at me when I arrive. It's never a good sign when the community is gathered outside. Inside a fifteen-year-old patient is fully dilated with her first baby, contracting three times every ten minutes. However, there's no engagement of the head and she's only approximately thirty weeks. She's obstructed, possibly a brow presentation, which occurs when the hard forehead is lined up to go through the pelvis first instead of the soft back of the head. Liaising with ARRA to get the permit, then realising it's night and we can't send the MSF ambulance due to security reasons, I organise for the BOH ambulance to be used, but then it's out of petrol, so we have to source petrol from somewhere in the middle of the night. We eventually get this all sorted. And we send her to the hospital in Gambella with two carers and two midwives. On arrival there, a tiny baby is born via c-section. Then another! No-one, including me, had picked up that the patient was carrying twins. I'm told the mother is doing well, but the babies – who weighed just 900 grams and 600 grams – did not survive.

Tuesday: A woman presents at the clinic, fully dilated with the baby's head visible. She gives birth to the baby within fifteen minutes of arriving. I am lucky to catch the healthy baby boy as he comes flying into the world. Later today I saw my first ever twins delivery with a footling breech, 2.5 kilogram and 2.6 kilogram twin boys. A good outcome was getting them all prepared for emergency transfer and the footling breech just came out beautifully, followed forty-five minutes later by his brother who came out headfirst much better. No issues. It's a good day.

Wednesday: It's late at night and I'm called out to a transverse lie (where the baby is positioned horizontally across the uterus rather than vertically) in a nineteen-year-old patient. This is her third baby. She is 7 centimetres dilated and when I do a vaginal exam, a tiny hand grasps my finger. As amazing as it is, this is not normal. The woman needs a c-section urgently, and she's transported to Gambella for one. Had the woman been left in the community, she would have lost the baby, developed sepsis, and likely died soon after.

Thursday: A nineteen-year-old woman is admitted after a suicide attempt. She is approximately ten weeks pregnant, comes from a broken family and has no support. After talking with the patient, the medical team and the authorities at MSF, it's decided that the woman will have an abortion at her request. I'm the one who gives the patient the abortion drug and I'm the one who gets to see her smile with relief.

Friday: We deliver two babies within one hour. The first woman needs a vacuum delivery requiring an episiotomy and sutures. The 'vacuum' is a glass bottle with a plastic suction cap attached to something that resembles a bike pump. The contraption looks like an ancient, barbaric – and quite phallic – apparatus. The second woman comes in with the baby's head already visible and delivers minutes later. A boy and a girl.

Saturday: I only worked a half-day in the morning, but I'm called back to the clinic after dinner to help out in the ED. A young woman has been stabbed in the chest. She has a 2-centimetre laceration and possible internal bleeding. She does not look well because she is not well. We try to stabilise and save her; there is no option for a blood transfusion or surgery, which she needs. We believe the small 2-centimetre stab wound punctured her heart and she dies at 8 pm. We are unable to save her. The wailing begins soon after and within ten minutes the body is gone, wrapped up and taken by the family. There was nothing we could do.

Sunday: It's my day off and I head to my favourite bar in the village for quite some time, not knowing tragedy has struck the extended family of the owners. Two days ago, three members of the family were murdered by people from across the border. A wife, her husband and their three-month-old baby were killed. Their eight-year-old managed to escape, but the killers took the three-year-old with them. Never to be seen again. This is what living near a civil war means: families killed, toddlers taken, orphans made.

It's a horrific story, and I'm taken to the family in mourning to pay my respects. In a *tukul* with mud on the walls and cow skins on the ground, an infant sleeps in the corner while the men and women gather to honour those they've lost. I am ushered in, feeling completely overwhelmed and so intrusive, and the women start touching my hands and bowing and I realise I am somehow a symbol of hope. I am not intruding, but paying my respects to a mourning family and they are appreciative of such respect. It is incredibly humbling.

I am told that if women start coming up to me in public and hold my hand, it is not aggression; they are showing respect for the respect I gave them. I have to be mindful of this because imagine if some stranger comes up to you and holds your hand, speaking in a language you don't understand and you dismiss them even though they have been through such pain.

I have been asked how I cope with the suffering I see as a RAN and MSF midwife. In a way, I don't. I've become very good at disassociating. At work, I put on my nurse mask and do my job. That's all I can do. When the problems of the world seem too huge to handle, I think of the classic starfish story: an old man sees a young boy throwing starfish back into the sea from a beach where tens of thousands of them lie. The man looks at the boy and tells him he won't be able to make a difference. The boy picks up another starfish, looks at the man and throws it back into the ocean. 'It sure made a difference to that one,' he says.

* * *

A week after I sent her for a c-section at Gambella, the nineteen-year-old with the transverse lie returned to Pugnido with her newborn baby. We made a difference to her.

I try to focus on the good. There was a lot of good here. In the village, the kids would see me coming and dared each other to get close to me; the six-year-olds with the toddlers on their hips came up to have a closer look, only to have the toddlers look at me and scream, then the six-year-old would take two steps back and the baby would stop. Again two steps forward and screaming. I never knew I was so scary! I wrote in my diary, 'I feel like an albino hippopotamus in a land of floating gazelles.'

I looked so different to them. But we had more in common than we knew. When I started to sing the 'ABCs', the kids took over and sang the rest. How they knew the entire English alphabet, I had no idea. My heart swelled. Something so familiar set within something so foreign.

One day I was walking to work from the compound when a woman stopped me and grabbed my hands. She spoke to me in language and blew/spat on my hands before putting her hands on my head and blowing some more on either side of my face, all the while speaking passionately in a language I did not understand. It was an unusual experience, but not a frightening or upsetting one. The woman was intense, but there was a strength and a calmness to her. She walked away from me as quickly as she had approached me, leaving me somewhat stunned in the street. A passer-by told me that I'd just been blessed by a Nuer woman.

I welcomed the blessing. It made me feel accepted; like I belonged in this place so far away from where I was born.

In the maternity ward, there were many moments of joy. After delivering a baby boy in the birthing room, I followed the mother back to her bed in the maternity ward. I was carrying her son in my arms. There was a group of elders visiting the ward and they all started singing and clapping with big smiles, all wanting to see the baby. The extreme happiness of new life is infectious.

Another highlight came in the form of a patient who spoke perfect English. It was rare to be able to communicate with patients directly – instead of through a translator – so I relished the opportunity. The woman had a miscarriage, and her haemoglobin was extremely low, which wasn't good. She needed a blood transfusion, but (as you know by now) they weren't available and we'd been told that blood supplies were low at Gambella so they couldn't commit to giving her any. Fortunately, the bleeding stopped, and we treated her for anaemia by starting her on iron tablets and vitamin C. She was touch and go. I kept a close eye on her for three days and was relieved when she started to recover. With her on the mend, we had some fantastic chats. She told me about her life, and I told her about mine. It was extraordinary to think how we'd both ended up here in remote Ethiopia from different countries on different paths.

'Will you remember me?' she asked me on the day she was discharged.

'I will remember you. Will you remember me?' I asked back.

'You saved my life, I will remember you always,' she said.

Her words hit me in the heart. It was true, the team at the MSF clinic had saved her life – and now she could continue living. We embraced and she left.

It was these moments that reminded me why I was here.

Another chilling moment of pure joy in absolute chaos was in the middle of the night, getting called in at 2 am for a maternity emergency. A mother had delivered a healthy baby girl and had then started bleeding profusely. Her placenta was stuck. The team and I managed to save her by manually removing the placenta and giving appropriate medications. After the seriousness subsided and the mother was stable, I left the delivery room weary as the adrenaline was wearing off. A kind-eyed gentleman diligently waiting outside for any news of his wife and child stopped me. After I had told him the news that both were alive, he looked into my eyes and, holding my hands, he said graciously, 'You are an angel in the night.' Still to this day, the thought of this is like a warm embrace.

* * *

It was time to facilitate the handover from MSF to the Bureau of Health (BOH). After four months in Pugnido, the countdown was on and I was in full swing to hand over. On top of seeing patients, we were doing inventory of every item in the hospital. Every single pen, stapler, bed and tablet needed to be accounted for, and decisions needed to be made about what MSF would take to their new project and what would be left behind for the BOH team. I was learning a tonne about logistics just from being in the warehouse; every box of supplies was stamped with its country of origin. There were stamps from every corner of the world sitting in this remote storage shed in an Ethiopian national park. It was a reminder of how big MSF was, how far and wide they reached, and how hard they worked. Two years ago, this hospital was a shell of a building that feral dogs had taken over, now it was a fully functioning hospital. It still had the feral dogs, though.

Some members of the MSF team were starting to leave, and everyone had been given their final contracts. I would be leaving in February. To where? I wasn't sure. Hopefully to another posting in Ethiopia; I'd heard whispers of a role at the Kule/Tierkidi/Nguenyyiel refugee camps north of Pugnido.

I was sitting under a huge tree in the Pugnido 1 camp writing down a list of all the things I still needed to do for the handover. It was a 'cool' 33 degrees that day and people had jackets on! I'd just given one of the Nuer translators, Jeremiah, a pen. He was so grateful for the gift and immediately started writing things down on an old, withered piece of paper he pulled from his back pocket. He was forty-two years old, he said, pointing to his greying hair. Jeremiah told me he was constantly trying to improve his English, so when he sat on a brick beside me, he pointed to it and asked what it was called. I told him and he wrote it down with his new pen.

'White is good,' he said, pointing to the white paper he was writing on. 'If you write on black, you don't see.'

As he told me this, his mouth formed a cheeky grin. And then trying to write on his skin, he was pointing out that my white skin could be written on and his black skin could not. I smiled at Jeremiah, who thanked me once more for the pen, told me not to forget his name, and left me sitting under the huge tree.

* * *

It was 1 am. I'd just fallen asleep after a farewell bonfire for our MSF expat doctor who was returning home to Copenhagen – a tradition when someone leaves – when the radio crackled. Down the broken line, I heard the words 'maternity emergency, 1.2 kilogram baby' and 'coming in from ARRA'. I was exhausted but managed to get up. There's nothing quite like an emergency to force you awake after forty-five minutes of sleep. I got dressed, woke up the driver and staggered to the hospital. When I arrived, I was pleased to see that the mother was well and the baby was in pretty good shape – all things considered. The baby, however, was hypoglycaemic. I managed to give him some glucose, put in a cannula and nasal gastric tube and snuggled him in with his mum to start kangaroo care.

'What about the other one?' someone asked.

'The other what?'

'The other baby!'

'Oh bloody hell.' The pile of cloths on the bed was not a pile of cloths at all, but a twin. There was a second baby weighing 1.3 kilograms. We administered the same treatment for the second child. Then both babies were stable and snuggled up. They were so tiny. If they survived the night, they would be transported to Gambella Hospital first thing in the morning, where MSF Spain had recently set up a neonatal department of sorts, the first of its kind in this region. They survived the night and with one bub tucked in the top of the mother and the other in the grandmother's top, they were transferred on the three and a half to four-hour hellish trip to Gambella. I found out later they were doing well.

Handing over to the BOH staff was a challenge, and would have been a near comical event if it wasn't so important. But it all went ahead and we were making progress with baby steps. The bosses were in their early thirties, doctors who had been pushed to management. Most were obstructive and defiant, but some were kind and trying to do their best for the patients. Daily, I would seek out Nahom, the kindest of all, and we would joke about how many fires needed to be put out in management to ensure a smooth handover.

The time had come, the Médecins Sans Frontières flag had been taken down, and we'd officially handed the hospital over to BOH and health posts to ARRA. There was a finality to it: I knew I would never be here again. It was heartbreaking. A concerned dad came up to me in our final days and asked us why we were leaving, that we were needed there, pointing down to his toddler son with an arm in a cast. He asked when and how to take the cast off as there were now limited services for refugees. I couldn't tell him, I had no idea how the service would be run after we left and all I could do was hope this toddler got the care he needed. It was so hard to leave.

Enjoying a wine with Dad at the Laggan Pub, our local and my favourite. Many a beverage has been shared here.

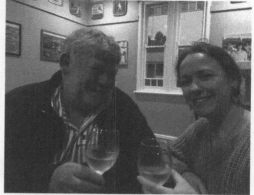

Right: My mentor, grandma, friend and most admired person, Mardi.

Below: Sitting with Mum in the sun at Manly Wharf in Sydney, catching up after another trip.

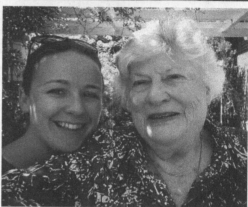

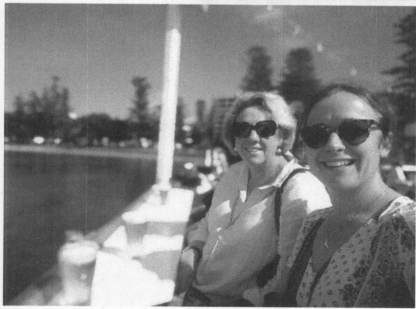

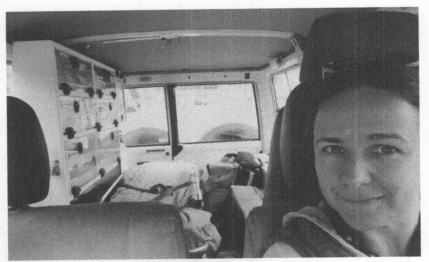

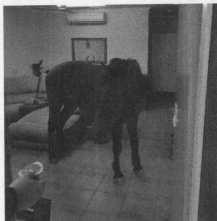

Above: RAN life, driving the troopie ambulance.

Left: Sunshine the stubborn horse in my house, Northern Territory.

Below: This is the way I love the outback, camping in perfect spots like this with friends, food and fire.

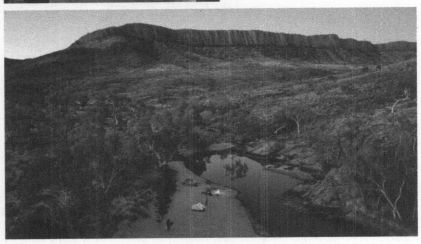

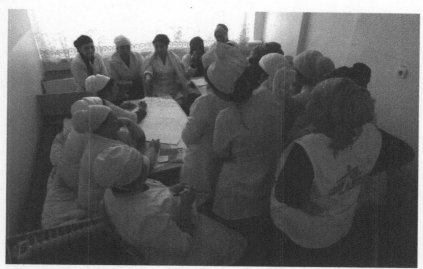

Above: Training
the nurses in
Kulob, Tajikistan,
on safe needle
use. Ozodamo, in
the MSF shirt, is
running the show.

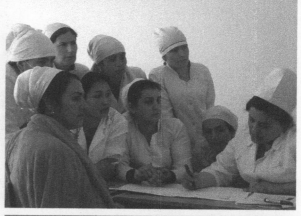

Middle: Nurses
being taught. The
brightly coloured
dressing gowns
were a common
item of clothing
in Kulob to keep
warm.

Right: Playing
in the snow in
Tajikistan, wearing
my pristine white
MSF t-shirt. Later,
in Ethiopia, they
were never this
white again.

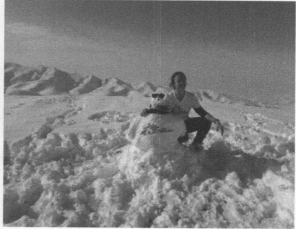

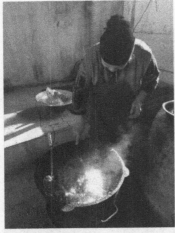

Left: It must be Friday in Tajikistan – here is our wonderful cook, Delaram, preparing *osh* in the woodshed.

Middle: A typical outing in Kulob, Tajikistan – MSF staff sitting on the floor with a banquet of food in the centre.

Below: The infamous game of *buzkashi* in Tajikistan. Somewhere in that chaos is a headless goat.

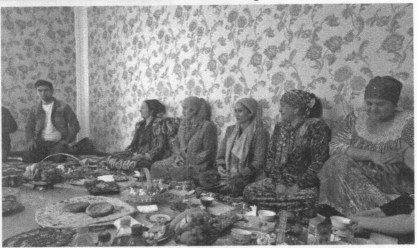

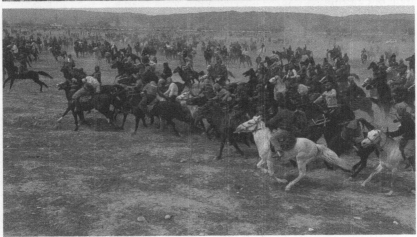

One of my favourite photos of the Tierkidi maternity unit in Ethiopia, soon after we opened.

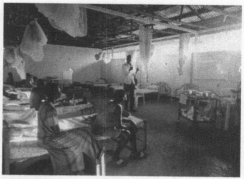

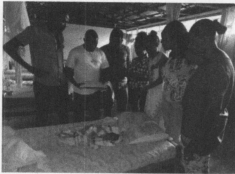

Here are some of the team during handover in Tierkidi's new 24-hour maternity unit.

Emilie the training doll. The women in the maternity unit loved her – she made many people smile.

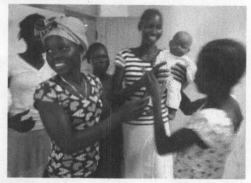

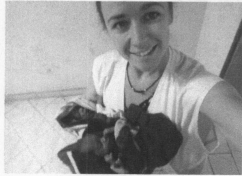

Newborn twins about to be transported from Pugnido to Gambella for care.

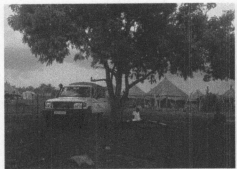

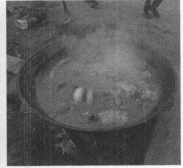

Top left: Break time in Nguenyyiel refugee camp.

Top right: Try anything once, horse innard stew, delicious. Would you try it?

Left: The junction near Kule on the way to Tierkidi. I had many coffees here.

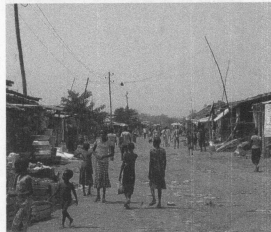

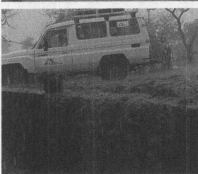

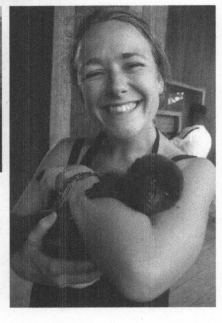

Above: The wet season begins, and there is a slight waterfall problem at the maternity unit.

Right: Meeting the friendly baby orphan spider monkeys of the Amazon.

Loving life
with the three
champagne limit
in the geothermal
sea baths, Húsavik,
Iceland.

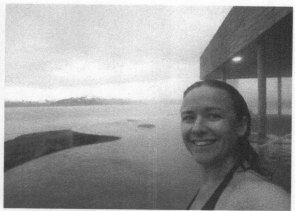

The epic views
on the O Trek,
Torres del Paine,
Patagonia.

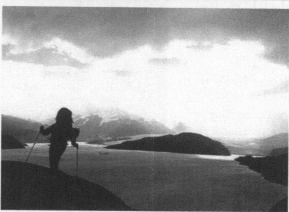

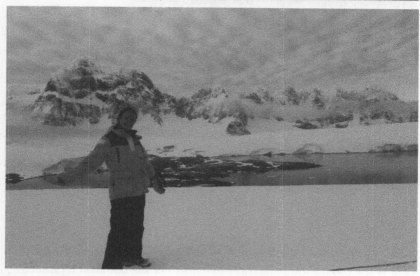

How did I get here? The raw beauty of Antarctica.

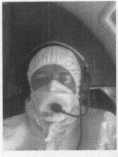

Above: In full PPE, transporting Covid-positive patients on the RFDS plane during the summer months in Central Australia.

Right: Inside the RFDS PC-12 plane, setting up the ventilator on the way to a patient in the middle of the night.

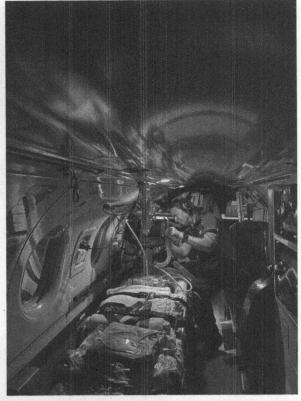

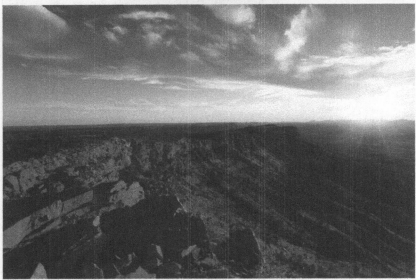

One of the thousands of pictures I've taken of the outback, a perfect sunset over the MacDonnell Ranges near Alice Springs.

CHAPTER SIX

Tierkidi, Ethiopia

'I feel like an albino hippopotamus in a land of
floating gazelles.'

– Diary entry

It was mango season in Ethiopia. Every corner had a mango stall, every kid had a sticky, yellow stain on their face, and every day I treated myself to the tropical fruit. Ten mangos cost 20 birr, which was 90 Aussie cents. The locals didn't cut them open with a knife, but ate them by biting the skin off and gobbling the juicy flesh down to the core. It was joyous to watch, and the smell of the ripe mangos reminded me of tropical holidays. I'd arrived in Kule in March – the hottest month of the year – and I was sleeping with a wet sarong draped over me and the fan on full blast beside me. The heat was brutal.

It was 17 kilometres from Kule to Tierkidi, the refugee camp where I'd be working. I lived in a compound with frogs in the shower, three cats, a puppy and two dogs named Double and Trouble. I also shared the expat compound with two Dutch nurses and a Dutch project coordinator, a Kenyan medical team leader and lab tech, a Rwandan doctor, a Japanese doctor, a Brazilian anthropologist, an English midwife, an Icelandic mental health officer and an American epidemiologist. We were a six-continent party, which is basically a full house because you can't come from the seventh continent. Sitting around the kitchen table, we bonded over the universal language of food. The Kenyans ate with their hands, I shovelled food into my mouth quickly alongside the Brit, and the Japanese doctor took eloquent, tiny mouthfuls from her organised plate. It was noted that we were all a long way from home, and there are many ways to do one thing.

It's always an adjustment when arriving in a new place. My sanctuary is where the fairy lights are. When moving to my next assignment, I always take fairy lights with me. They comfort me, they warm me, they make me feel safe. For me, arriving at a new location means making the most of the situation. And not having any expectations. As soon as you have expectations and they're not met, you're disappointed. Take out the expectation then it's just like, oh sweet, this works.

* * *

I split my time between Kule, where I lived; Gambella, where I sometimes stayed and where my Pugnido team lived; Tierkidi, where we were opening a maternity unit; and Nguenyyiel, where we were operating and opening health posts. I learned that MSF treated more than 300,000 patients in the previous year in the different regions' refugee camps.

The short journey from my *tukul* home in Kule to work in Tierkidi took forty minutes because the roads were so terrible. Driving through Kule took fifteen minutes because we could only go 10 kilometres an hour on the bumpy dirt track. This was my favourite part of the trip, though. From the troopie, I loved to sit back and watch people going about their daily activities. I saw many women with giant sacks balanced on top of their heads. One woman had the sack and a teapot balanced perfectly on top of it. I saw groups of women filling up yellow jerry cans at the water point where children splashed about in whatever puddles they could find. I saw people going in and out of their homes, which were made of dried mud and surrounded by gardens and fences built with timber and tall dry grass. Some of the homes were painted on the outside, while others were left *au naturel*. Everything seemed clean and well-maintained. It was amazing to me that in this hot part of Ethiopia, some gardens were green and blooming.

There were people who sat outside their homes all day. I'd drive past them in the morning on my way to work, and ten hours later in the afternoon on my way home, they'd still be sitting in the exact same spot. Some of those people sold little trinkets in a pile on the ground in front of them. Others simply watched the world go by. One day we drove past a group of teenage boys with a speaker of some description blaring music across the area. The music was terrible but it was music, a universal language reminding me that no matter how far away you are from your home, music is still an important aspect of life wherever you are. Kids were dancing naked in the streets and teenagers were playing it cool in the shadows. It is the same the world over.

Once we made it through Kule, there was a checkpoint, and after that we hit the main road. It was tarred, so we could go a whopping 50 kilometres an hour. The speedy highway took us to 'The Junction', a busy area full of people, cars, shops, pool tables, music and tuk tuks, which were called *bajaj*. Kids rode bikes, women served tea on plastic tables and cooked bread in huge clay ovens, and men wore full suits in the sticky heat. The adults were all incredibly tall – at least six foot – and the kids were both shy and cheeky. Some kids spotted me in the troopie and yelled out, '*Nyakuawaja*', which translates to 'colourless person'.

'I wonder who they're referring to,' I looked around sarcastically. I wrote again in my diary, 'I still feel like an albino hippo surrounded by floating gazelles.'

On our drive through Tierkidi, we passed the food ration collection point. It was closed that day so the area was empty. When it was open, it could take us ten minutes to get through the thick crowd in the car. A naked little boy ran across the road with his toy – a tyre rim and a stick. The driver playfully beeped the horn at him, and he ran quicker, his dusty bottom disappearing into a mud hut. The guards at the maternity ward greeted me with a handshake, and my day officially began …

The first time I arrived at the MSF clinic in Tierkidi to start my role, I was a sweaty mess. All I knew about the posting was that it involved helping to set up a new 24-hour maternity base for the camp's 100,000 and counting refugees.

I asked someone what the plan was. Their response was, 'Whatever you say, you're the boss!' I didn't like this answer very much so I went and found the project coordinator and asked him the same question. 'You're it. And you're late,' was his response.

Okay then! The plan, as I saw it, was to turn a shell of a building in the Tierkidi Refugee Camp into a functioning 24-hour maternity hospital as soon as possible, to service both Tierkidi and Nguenyyiel refugees. Kule already had its own well-functioning maternity unit. Fortunately the Kule team had recruited many of the midwives and I'd be interviewing three more that week in Addis Ababa. So I had staff, tick. I had shelter, tick. Electricity, not so much. Water, work in progress. Still under construction were the laundry, latrines, kitchen, sterilisation room, driver accommodation, generator shed and water supply plan. Oh, and we needed incentive staff, security staff, and above all we needed to implement a community awareness program to let people know we were there. No good having the service available if no-one knew about it.

The project seemed enormous because it was enormous. Oh yeah, and I had three months to do it. I didn't know where to begin, but I started anyway. Many phenomenal experiences and small wins with many frustrations summarised my day to day.

Heading to Addis Ababa for the planned interviews was first on my list of jobs. It was there I met Weyni, an excellent midwife and a gorgeous human. I'm sharing her stories of recent times and tribulations as every woman needs a voice and I have the privilege and permission to be hers.

* * *

Weyni was born in Tigray, Ethiopia. She had five sisters and a brother and her family were farmers. Her uncle's wife raised her. After she finished school she did a four-year midwifery degree, which she completed in 2014. She worked in the Somali region, then applied for an MSF job, which is when I met her in Addis Ababa. After a quick interview I wanted her on my team. She was kind, competent, caring and had a passion for women's health and midwifery. Accepting the job, she moved from the east of Ethiopia to the west and started work with me in Tierkidi. I was the only person she knew, but she quickly settled in and became a valued team member.

We celebrated the opening of the maternity hospital together and later my farewell. Since then we have remained in contact through social media. At the end of 2020 the country suffered civil unrest and the Tigray conflict erupted with Tigrayan people feeling unsafe across the country. Since then, Weyni has had no contact with her family.

She continued doing the work she loved at the maternity hospital in Tierkidi, but then police came to her home to arrest her, which she believed was because she was from Tigray. Fortunately she was at work and when she got home her neighbours warned her. She stayed with a friend and continued going to work, until it became too unsafe so she made the decision to flee. Through a South Sudanese friend who knew how to cross the border, she left for South Sudan. After a dangerous journey, mostly on foot through the African wilderness, with no food, no clean water and gunfire within earshot, she was able to reach Juba, where she found safe shelter with some other Tigray refugees. She still lives in Juba, unable to work as a midwife, and has opened a small shop selling knick-knacks to keep afloat. Weyni will not give up trying to find her family and is secure in Juba for now, but she does not know what her future will hold. She is my friend and I have so much respect for her. Weyni gave me permission to include her story here so she can be heard, to be one voice among the thousand of untold stories.

* * *

In addition to sixteen midwifery staff, I needed to hire twenty-six incentive staff – refugees from the area hired to work as cleaners, translators, laundry workers, kitchen staff, water carriers, sterilisation workers, and everything in between. Hiring the incentive staff wasn't a straightforward task. The HR manager told the 'zone leaders' that we'd be holding interviews in the maternity building for anyone with the relevant skills. On the day of the interviews, 300-plus people showed up. It was clear that most of them didn't know what jobs we were hiring for, but they were desperate for work. We tried to see as many people as we could, but the crowd outside grew restless and pushed the gate open to storm inside. Security had to step in. At no point was I in harm's way, but I was shaken by the desperation of the people who simply wanted to work.

The next time we did the interviews, we learned from our mistake and asked for only women to apply. We already had a male-heavy midwifery team, so we decided to open up the incentive work opportunity to the women of the camp.

Incredibly, with the collective effort of everyone involved – the Kule team, the Gambella team and all in between – we managed to work together and make substantial progress with opening the unit. The equipment was 70 per cent organised and the pharmacy was on track. Medical forms were mostly printed and I had the warehouse staff stapling thousands of papers together for me on a Saturday, which didn't make me very popular. In the meantime the builders were finishing construction of the sterilisation shed, laundry and kitchen, and I was organising the medical aspect of emergency boxes, registration books and neonatal resus training programs. I even managed to make a four-page orientation book for the new staff. Although I wasn't sure if this was for me or them!

The week leading up to the opening of the maternity ward was chaos. No, that's not quite right. It was CHAOTIC.

Six days before we opened, we managed to successfully finish allocating and training the twenty-six (female) incentive workers.

Four days before we opened, a truckload of essential equipment arrived – mattresses, delivery beds, basic furniture and the pharmacy order.

Three days before opening, the staff and I were frantically setting up all the equipment, allocating rooms for assessment: antenatal, labouring, delivering, postnatal, storage, rainbow room and office/pharmacy.

Two days before, the electricity was turned on.

One day before, the electricity failed and was turned off.

On the day of the opening, there were three staff rostered on and ... not a single patient. Thankfully, because the generator still wasn't working, so there was no electricity in the building. But we did it! The staff were set up with head torches and spent the first night there. Due to security reasons I wasn't allowed to join them. But we did it, we set up a semi-functioning maternity hospital – and even though there was still an unbelievable amount of work to do, it was 'ready'. We'd installed a maternity department in a refugee camp.

The next day, our first patient came in at thirty-six weeks pregnant and with malaria. The second patient was a septic abortion, and the third was a sexual and gender-based violence (SGBV) survivor. Community awareness about us was growing and the need clearly evident. Like any new department, it came with trials and tribulations, failures and successes. We had it all.

Within that first week we changed the entire layout of two of the rooms to have better patient flow. We had to install strict medication stock counts: if we ran out it was an ordeal to get more – at least a four-hour round trip. Electricity was a constant battle – no matter how hard I worked to get it fixed, most nights the midwives were working by head torch.

A week after the maternity hospital officially opened for business, an opening ceremony was held. Or, rather, our ridiculously busy and hard-working team were 'asked' to hold an opening ceremony on top of their actual jobs. All the big players in the region attended: the United Nations High Commission for Refugees (UNHCR), the International Rescue Committee (IRC), the Administration for Refugees and Returnee Affairs (ARRA) and of course Médecins Sans Frontières. This was more for them than it was for us. A cake was baked, songs were sung and a ribbon was cut. There was dancing and singing, and everyone involved was congratulated. It all felt perfunctory to me, no doubt because

I was annoyed about us having to organise the whole thing when we had real work to do.

I made eye-contact with Tesfahun, the midwife supervisor and my right-hand man, and gave a discreet eye-roll at the powerful men patting themselves on the back for a job they didn't do. If anyone deserved all the credit, it was Tesfahun. He was the backbone of the maternity hospital and had been invaluable in setting it up. We'd worked closely together, and he'd become a dear friend. He was the one who would continue the work, as I'd be leaving.

When I first arrived in Ethiopia it was interesting how many men were midwives. In Australia it's such a female-dominated industry, but there it is the opposite. It took some getting used to, having so many men around 'women's business', but it was just another thing to remind me I was not at home and there are so many ways to achieve the same results.

I leaned heavily on Tesfahun. He explained so many cultural nuances to me and gave me helpful tips. His bedside manner was so calm, caring and respectful, and his experience was invaluable. While I'm singing Tesfahun's praises, one of the best things about him was how he wasn't afraid of me. He told me when I was wrong and we worked on a solution together. We were a good team. While all the bureaucrats were eating cake, I thanked Tesfahun for all his hard work.

Then – as if they knew the timing was right – two women arrived in labour, and not long after, two babies were born. It was a christening of sorts; a wetting of the maternity ward's head. Now it felt real.

I felt real, too. When I first landed in Ethiopia, I was faking it until I made it. You can if you think you can. Now I didn't need to fake it (nearly as much). I didn't bat an eyelid when a kamikaze lizard flew from the ceiling during an SGBV consult, likewise when a snake slithered across the kitchen floor during dinner, or when I discovered bats in the postnatal room. It was totally normal for me to have two goats in the back of the troopie on the way to camp, and for those two goats to become dinner.

I poured my heart and soul into this project, giving every inch of energy, commitment and resilience I could muster. It became my world, and I was totally absorbed.

At lunch, I would be served a meal in a black plastic bag, and I ate it with my hands, as is the custom. It's also a sign of respect to feed other people, an affectionate tradition called *gursha*, so I got used to having food shoved into my mouth by the midwives on days when I was too busy to sit down to eat. My usual lunchtime order depended on what was available on the day and could include spicy meat, cabbage, egg, a cheese-like substance or goat. It changed daily, but it was always delicious. The meal, a 2-litre bottle of water and a mango cost me 50 birr (AU$2.30). I might have grown used to eating with my hands (and from other people's hands), but I still flinched at how cheap things were.

I preferred the Ethiopian food over the Nuer food. Some of my Nuer team members would eat a millet porridge with a stew of some kind and one dish I couldn't bear – a green (not sure what vegie it was) soup thing the consistency of raw egg white. I was not a fan, but apart from that the food was generally delicious with unique flavours and textures.

At night in the Kule compound there was less variety, but the food was cooked over hot coals daily, including yummy homemade bread. Dinner was generally a carbohydrate overload of rice, pasta, potatoes and bread.

* * *

In Gambella I met Paul, the new MSF logistician from America, who was a jack of all trades, master of none.

He also happened to be a good-looking 33-year-old bloke. Suddenly, I was painfully aware of how devoid of romantic attention I was. I was quietly pleased to have someone attractive to admire and have a cheeky flirt with. It was a harmless distraction, nothing more.

Truth be told, Paul was a bit of an arsehole. He was borderline rude to most people, but lovely to me. He intrigued me. Plus, somehow, he had access to really good treats and drinks. I'm not saying you can win me over with a hot toddy, but … it worked. Covered in amniotic fluid and mud I would head to Gambella to pick up supplies, and Paul would welcome me to the compound with a hot toddy, calm music, an actual hot shower and a delicious home-cooked meal. I was in. The attraction turned physical and I spent more time in Gambella than Kule in those final months. It was a welcome distraction.

* * *

The first time I see the nomads, they're walking into the camp at Tierkidi with their donkeys. I'm mesmerised by them. The men carry long walking sticks and wear outfits that look like abayas with red tassels around the hems and the women carry babies on their backs, wearing more jewellery than clothes; jewellery decorates their necks, arms and abdomens. Long, flowing blue and white robes drape over them. They speak some form of Arabic and they walk with purpose and power. They are captivating and enthralling.

I discover the reclusive nomads are called the Falata and are a collection of Arab tribal communities who migrated from western Africa to greater Sudan. Today, they rear herds of cattle and walk from Nigeria through Chad and Sudan, into South Sudan and across the Gambella region of Ethiopia, before turning around and making the year-long journey back to where they started. They have no home, all they have is what they carry. They have no passports or formal identity; on paper, they do not exist.

Depending on who you ask, the Falata are either considered sacred or dirty. Some say if you harm a Falata, you will face the wrath of the spirits; that's why they go undisturbed by the tribes they come across on their journey. Others refuse to eat at places were Falata frequent because they sleep with their cows and never wash.

One day, a group of Falata women unexpectedly showed up at the clinic. This was so unusual as they have their own survival skills and medical practices. As the wary clinic staff tried to communicate with them, I tried to make them feel as comfortable as possible. They clearly didn't trust me – they appeared terrified by me, especially when I made the mistake of reaching out to touch a shoulder as a way to show comfort. The woman flinched and scuttled away, so I stood back at a distance to reassure them. We were trying to find out what they needed. One of the women had a very infected cut on her leg, which could be treated with antibiotics and a tetanus injection to potentially save her life. But trying to explain this, gain consent and give Westernised treatments was nearly impossible. Despite a series of charades and kind smiles, they left with no treatment. I could only hope their own remedies saved the woman from sepsis.

* * *

At one point an anthropologist visited the Nguenyyiel camp. He witnessed some severe neglect in the area, and to investigate what the health needs were, we organised a mobile clinic. Staff who were happy to sacrifice their Sunday went out to this area to set up the clinic under a giant mango tree, complete with a doctor, a nurse, a medication dispensary and a registration staff member. It was quick, efficient and so impressive. I walked through the community in a team of three to communicate with the help of our translator that we had a mobile clinic up under the big tree, and that if anybody was sick or pregnant they should go and see them. During these conversations, sitting in the dirt surrounded by people, we would ask how many deaths or births there had been in the area. We asked them how and where they got their food and water, how many people lived in their tents, how long they had been there, how long it took them to get there, and why they had left South Sudan. We quickly found out they only had the clothes on their backs, the tents were small with five or more people living in them, with a dirt floor, no blankets and no jerry cans to collect water, which was more than an hour's walk away. The toilet buildings were dilapidated so open defecation was everywhere. The ground was quite spongy so I could only imagine what would unfold when the rainy season hit. With no provisions, no protection, no escape, it was a disaster waiting to happen.

The medics under the big tree saw sixty-one patients in an hour. That's one a minute. It was remarkable. The need for medical help was so apparent. There was a real sense of the camp teetering on the edge of no return. Without intervention, a deadly outbreak would most certainly be the reality. With intervention? We could only hope.

I became a clown, running around with the kids as they mimicked everything I did – jumping up and down, running and hopping around, touching my nose, sticking out my tongue. The kids grew in number and it was fun, exhausting and humbling. The smiles and giggles were so infectious – these kids, the poorest of the poor, had so much joy.

I suddenly realised we had bottles of water in the car, which would be a lifeline, something to carry water in. I spoke with the medical team leader about giving the bottles to them. He was concerned for our safety because there weren't enough for all of them. We ended up throwing them from the safety of the troopies and left in a cloud of dust with the kids shoving and pushing to get the life-saving bottles to transport water. It was heartbreaking.

* * *

After a week in Nguenyyiel, I sat down with the camp's zonal leaders and elders under the big mango tree to listen to their concerns and needs. I had the joyful job of telling the group that there was a new 24-hour maternity department where they could go to birth safely, and a new medical outpost in the refugee camp to come. The news was welcomed with a round of applause. And many questions. Who can go there? When could they go there? Where is it? Is it free?

The experience of working in crisis management and identification was entirely new to me, and utterly thrilling. Responding to an evolving situation is scary, but there's an immense satisfaction as well. You can see first-hand the difference you're making in real time. I knew without a doubt that the work the team and I did in a single week in Nguenyyiel would save lives. Lots of them. The scale of impact you could have here was huge. Yet, realistically, for every life we saved there were hundreds more not being saved.

* * *

Back in Tierkidi, it had been a month since the maternity ward opened. In that time, we'd seen everything: the extreme, the unusual and the ordinary. There were SGBV cases, pre-term deliveries, stillborns, neonates that thrived against the odds, post-partum haemorrhages, terminations, and a very interesting case of a newborn patient who was unable to open his mouth wider than a fingertip. He couldn't cry or breastfeed. I queried whether he had tetanus or a congenital abnormality. Devastatingly, his chances of survival were slim. We had one heartbreaking maternal death in this time, from pre-eclampsia. The woman presented to the maternity unit too late. We couldn't save her.

After spending a morning checking in on things at the Nguenyyiel health posts, I got back to the maternity ward to find a room full of patients, without any notes, arrival times, observations or diagnostics. I had no idea what was happening with each patient – and it seemed no-one else did either. Bloody hell. The constant battle of paperwork is not my forte but there is a need for it and simple notes on timing, observations, diagnosis and treatment given are essential when it comes to ongoing healthcare. It appeared the team and I were forgetting the basics.

It was something we really needed to improve on, and I told the team as much. The importance of paperwork was reinforced to me once again at a meeting with ARRA and UNHCR about the registration of babies. In the time when Tierkidi was without a maternity department, babies were delivered in tents and paperwork (obviously) wasn't done for them. Now, there were 714 unregistered babies in the region that were known of, and no doubt many more that were unknown. Without registration, these babies wouldn't get a ration card as they grew up, which meant no food or school.

'How am I meant to feed my family? What am I meant to do?' cried a mother holding her unregistered, approximately nine-month-old baby.

I didn't have an answer for her. All we could do was add names to a list of unregistered babies and give that to the authorities to figure out a way to get them registered. It wasn't enough. I knew that, and the mother in tears knew it too. But we were just cogs in the wheel.

It was horrific. And it was all because some bloody forms weren't filled out.

It wasn't lost on me that the reason I left Tajikistan was because it felt like all I did was paperwork, and now all I wanted was for paperwork to be done.

A pregnant woman arrived at the maternity ward in active labour – as many of them do. She delivered a baby boy without any issues, and instead of a placenta another baby was delivered, which was a surprise for us and for the mother – she was having twins. The second baby was a breech presentation and much more difficult to deliver. I'd been taught to use a hands-off approach, with the understanding that any downward pressure could deflect the head and therefore impact it in the mother's birth canal. The baby eventually came out. When he did, he wasn't the colour he should have been. We performed a full resus. There was no response. The baby had died, and I believe it was because I took too long to deliver him. I was shattered. It was hard not to feel responsible when I was the one delivering the babies, even though these things were out of my control.

When I told the family that the second baby hadn't made it, they said, '*Goer*', which means 'good' in Nuer.

'No, not good. The baby has died. I'm so sorry,' I tried to explain with help of a translator, thinking they'd misunderstood me.

'*Goer*,' they insisted. They appeared nonchalant about one of their babies dying – later I learned why: to survive one baby was much easier than surviving two. Infant and child morbidity and mortality were very high under the age of five.

It wasn't the response I was used to, but it was the reality here.

As I was leaving the clinic for the day, a nine-year-old boy arrived with internal injuries. He had been raped by his neighbour. This, too, was the reality here. I took him and his carer to Kule health camp emergency section to be looked after there.

When I finally got home, I had a little cry and decompressed by watching an episode of *Grey's Anatomy*, my usual go-to when I need my brain to disengage. It had been a shit day, but I couldn't dwell on it for too long because I needed to get up in the morning and do it all over again.

A much-needed morale booster arrived in a cardboard box. The sender's address read, 'From: Mardi'. The package was full of tiny beanies which Mardi's friends had knitted for the premmie babies. The beanies were a rainbow of colours and seeing them made my heart happy. I could imagine her rallying the troops and organising the whole thing. Bless her. It was a kind gesture – and one everyone was grateful for – but a box of beanies didn't stretch very far here. The need was so great. This was a momentary band-aid, but it was a kind band-aid and it was better than nothing. Plus, the babies did look adorable in the beanies.

It felt like ages since I'd had a straightforward, stress-free, healthy delivery. After the breech birth where the twin died, I was hoping for a healthy delivery soon. I'm a midwife, that hankering comes with the territory. It probably goes without saying, but delivering a baby is an extraordinary rush. It never gets old. Mothers often talk about the intense emotions they feel when they see their baby for the first time.

Midwives feel the miracle of birth, too, albeit on a much lighter scale. Being a midwife is a job – there's no denying it's hard work – but it's also a very special thing to be able to help bring new life into the world.

It's not just about the new life, either. Seeing a woman become a mother, and a man become a father, is an incredible thing to witness. Birth is transformative. It's also vulnerable. Often, women don't recognise themselves in the birthing room. They disassociate from society's expectations of them, they stop playing the part of the elegant woman or the perfect partner, and they become the most raw version of themselves. It's instinctual and animalistic. Another force takes over entirely. There are howling noises, blood, sweat, and – often – shit. It happens.

To be in the room for such a powerful moment – and to see first-hand what the human body is capable of – is a privilege. There's nothing like delivering a healthy baby. It's the best part of the job, and the thought of it keeps me going on the hardest of days.

I got my wish: a woman arrived at the maternity ward fully dilated. She'd come in after a busy day – the ward had been full all morning and no-one had had a chance to restock the equipment. We didn't have any sterile delivery packs to use for the delivery, so I gloved up and made do with the string from a surgical mask (in lieu of cord clamps) and a clean razor that seemed to come out of nowhere. My makeshift delivery kit would have to do the trick.

The membranes ruptured – and I was in the wrong place at the wrong time and got covered in meconium-stained liquid. It's essentially the baby's first stool, but unlike later faeces, it's made of materials ingested in the uterus: intestinal epithelial cells, lanugo, mucus, amniotic fluid, bile and water.

Meconium liquid can be a sign of foetal distress, so I was relieved when a baby boy came out screaming and weighing a healthy 3.3 kilograms. Huge! The mother let out a slight cough and delivered the placenta. As soon as it came out, I knew it was unusual. After suturing a small tear on the mother I stood up to inspect the placenta more closely. What I found was fascinating. There was a twin, approximately eighteen weeks gestation, and another hard mass in the placenta, which I guessed was a third child. The twin wasn't decomposed, so I assumed they didn't die in the womb, but all their nutrients went to the surviving baby. The other baby mustn't have been compatible with life, so they never grew.

Later I found out vanishing twin syndrome is the loss of a developing baby early in a multiple pregnancy. The syndrome is typically diagnosed by ultrasound – where an early ultrasound shows a twin pregnancy and then the next ultrasound shows only one baby developing normally alongside a blighted ovum – so in places where ultrasounds aren't accessible, the condition goes undiagnosed. The reasons why vanishing twin syndrome develops aren't well understood. It doesn't happen because of anything the mother did or didn't do. It just happens.

Most commonly, the vanishing twin is absorbed by the mother's body so that there is no evidence of the twin at the time of birth. So it's pretty rare to see one vanishing twin after a delivery – let alone a possible two. Looking at the mum cradling her newborn son in her arms, I was in awe of the human body.

I was also still covered in liquid. One of the incentive workers noticed me, giggled and took my vest off me to wash it in the laundry. When they brought it back to me later in the day, it was whiter than it had ever been. They took such pride in getting things perfectly clean. Their clothes were always impeccably clean, colourful and immaculate. Not a stain or crease in sight. I really don't know how they got things so immaculate when water was scarce, soap was a luxury and flooring was dirt.

* * *

The weather was changing in Ethiopia. Later, in the compound, I was sitting outside having a beer with my housemates when the first storm hit. It had been so calm – too calm. Then, out of nowhere, there was a clap. The wind blew so hard that I was sure the trees were going to take off, and the rain fell so heavily that it looked like a solid curtain of water pelting down. The wind and the rain together was deafening. I sculled my beer and retreated to my room. Water sprayed onto my face through the high flyscreen that surrounded my small *tukul* while I was lying on my bed. It was going to be a long night.

The rains had indeed arrived, bringing with them grey skies and dramatic lightning. When the storms rolled in at work, it was impossible to have a conversation in the maternity ward because the rain was so relentlessly loud on the corrugated tin roof. It was deafening. The array of animals finding shelter from the rain led to a few concerns in the unit. Also, we almost flooded unexpectedly. Water gushed down the hill and poured over the clinic entrance in torrents. We frantically shovelled dirt and mud to stop it going inside. Fortunately we had a moat-like drainage system and the water never went inside this time.

I woke up to giant puddles on the drive from Kule to Tierkidi. Just when I was starting to get to know which potholes to brace for, the rain arrived and added a few more to my mental list. I didn't know how many more times I would drive this stretch of road. My end of mission date was looming, and I was working on a handover for my successor, a woman named Isla from Namibia. Plans were also being made for the international staff living in Kule and Gambella and working in Tierkidi to move to the tent city that was being built in the latter. We all had bets on when the tent city would actually open. Apparently, one of the tents blew away in the previous night's storm, so the chances of being moved there within the week were slim. It was high stakes: there was a carton of beer on the line (which cost AU$16.80).

We were discussing the bet at a Friday night MSF party in Gambella with the Operations Centre team from MSF Spain. I also learned of their incredible neonatal work at Gambella hospital – we now had somewhere safe to send the premature babies. This was a huge accomplishment. It was nice to see some new faces from MSF Spain and MSF Amsterdam, socialising and working so well together.

Back at work, I wrote a 4000-word handover document for Isla. It was a bittersweet process. I felt apprehensive about leaving something I'd helped to build out of nothing and had poured my heart and soul into. It was also a proud moment, looking back on all that we'd achieved. As I wrote I remembered there were some things I wouldn't miss – like the constant battle to keep equipment sterilised using the autoclave (a wild machine that required a steady coal supply to run). But the fact that I knew how to sterilise equipment using the autoclave was amazing. So, too, was my ability to source coal at a pinch at five o'clock on a Friday afternoon when the incentive staff tell me they're about to run out. I included in the notes to Isla how best to avoid this situation, but if it arose how to acquire the coal.

A new round of MSF workers had arrived to take over from those of us leaving, and their eyes were wide with awe. Or maybe it was fear? Or a substantial case of 'what the hell have I got myself into?' Either way, I knew it wouldn't last long.

I was showing one of the new nurses the maternity unit while running around simultaneously checking on patients, answering questions, filling out paperwork and talking in broken language. Suddenly a traditional birth attendant came rushing in holding a brand-new preterm baby. She was small and barely breathing. After some time the team and I were able to stabilise the baby. Back to the orientation for the nurse, and she was staring at me. A realisation hit: I am Will. When I first arrived in Ethiopia at my Pugnido posting, I remember I stared at Will, the nurse and medical team leader, and was amazed at the ease with which he worked. He was in total control; he knew everyone by name and everything that needed doing, and he spoke in broken language. What took me hours now took me minutes. After nine months in Ethiopia, I was that person now. It had been incredibly varied – the lows were desperately low and the highs were tremendous. It was a rollercoaster but ultimately I would not have changed a thing. Opening a 24-hour maternity hospital in a refugee camp was my biggest accomplishment to date.

I had to remind myself this was just a job, that there was always a leaving date and I couldn't stay. Even though my heart and soul had gone into the place, I held on to the hope that the work we had done would continue. Tesfaran assured me it would.

It was time to work out my next plans. And it was certainly not lost on me how privileged and fortunate I was – I had a choice whether to stay or go. I could leave at any time and go back to my world of abundance, of opportunity, education and a loving supportive family, surrounded by health care and security.

During my last few days in Kule – before moving out to spend a week in Gambella – I was at the office, tying up loose ends and getting ready for Isla's arrival. I hadn't met Isla or even spoken to her directly, but I felt weirdly connected to her. For the past two weeks, I'd been busily working to make her life as easy as possible when she got here. I was excited to be handing over to her, and eager to meet the person who would be following on with the work. Isla had been meant to arrive the day before, but I was told she'd missed her flight. No bother, I still had two weeks in the country, so another day wasn't going to hurt.

The office phone rang, I answered it, and what I was told crushed me. Isla missed her flight because she was in a car accident on the way to the airport. She did not survive.

Isla wasn't delayed, she was dead. The woman I'd been waiting for wasn't coming.

I dealt with death on a daily basis, I saw it up close, but I'd learned to distance myself from it. Even though Isla was miles away when she died and I'd never met her, her death hit me hard. It stopped me in my tracks. This would have been her first MSF assignment. I could imagine the emotions she would have been feeling on her way to the airport: fear, excitement, a sense of purpose. It hurt to know that all those emotions would have come to an abrupt end.

Later that day in Gambella, the project coordinator, Emma, came to find me. She knew about the accident and was a great comfort, allowing me time to process and comprehend what had happened. We discussed the project and the impact this death would have on it and the possibility of me staying longer until we found a replacement. There was a lot to be discussed, but in the end I realised my time was up. It was time to go home.

* * *

The tent city in Tierkidi was almost a mythological place at this point. It had been talked about since I'd arrived in Ethiopia, but I didn't think I'd actually get to experience it before I left. It had been a long time coming, made longer by the storm season that turned the tent city into a flood plain. In the end, I got to spend a total of one night in a tent there. The new team would move to Tierkidi in the coming weeks after I left.

A party was held to celebrate the opening of the tent city. It felt wrong to me. There was music, food and fun. The MSF team were outside and we were all making noise and having a good time. Meanwhile, we were in the refugee camp residents' backyard. We were moving into their space – where they'd fled to escape civil war – and we were chucking a party. I couldn't shake the feeling of it being disrespectful. Even though it should have been an enjoyable night, it wasn't for me.

It was a tricky balance to strike. On one hand, it was hard to celebrate things when you were surrounded by so much adversity. On the other, it was important and necessary to celebrate things when you were surrounded by so much adversity. Everyone needed to blow off steam and have moments of joy. It's what kept us going. As conflicted as I felt about the party, I knew the team needed it. It just could have been done differently.

My send-off went on for days. Incorporating the teams from Pugnido, Tierkidi, Kule, Gambella and Nguenyyiel, there were a lot of people to farewell, and I did what I could to tie up loose ends and put plans in place for the midwifery unit to stay afloat.

I took my midwifery team out to lunch at the Big Time Hotel in Gambella. There were speeches, gifts, tears and hugs. The team had bought me a handmade traditional green, gold and white Ethiopian dress. Weyni and some of the other girls ushered me away and dressed me up in this beautiful dress, a nice change from my cargo pants and dirty MSF t-shirt. I found it all very touching.

The best parting gift of all was a replacement. After Isla's sudden and tragic death, the MSF team scrambled to find someone else to take over from me. They found a woman named Jane from Kenya, a veteran MSF midwife. It was a relief to be handing over to someone with experience.

I only had six hours to hand over to Jane – it was a mammoth debrief, so she was understandably overwhelmed. But she was kind, gracious and eager to get stuck in, and I had full confidence in her. She was full of compliments for me and the team, taking time to learn the names of the staff and their responsibilities.

It all happened very quickly. Those final hours in the maternity unit were humbling, as I reflected on what it had been, to what it had become. A single shell of a building had been transformed into a fully functional 24-hour maternity unit, a safe, free space where women could come and deliver. There was a sterilisation shed, a good supply of coal for the autoclave, latrines, showers, a kitchen, a laundry, a generator shed, electricity. We had a water supply, although not from a tap – twice daily, eight or so Nuer women would gracefully appear with big, colourful 40-litre buckets filled with water on top of their heads and fill our buckets to keep a constant supply of water. We had wonderful staff: an incredible midwifery team and incentive workers who kept the place functioning. We had a pharmacy, beds, security and a fleet of cars and a bus to move the staff in and out of the camp daily for their shifts.

And of course we had patients, so many patients.

* * *

When we first opened we tried to encourage the community to come and attend for antenatal checks and birthing. Sadly we had a few cases come too late and mother and babies both died. This left the community wary of us and what we were doing, and they blamed us for the deaths. Understandable, but after many discussions and advocating with the village elders, we convinced them that women should come to the hospital when they first felt a baby pain to avoid tragic death. Our reputation improved and people continued coming from as far away as the furthest corner of the Nguenyyiel camp.

While debriefing with Jane on my last day, there were two deliveries. I watched one of the midwives catch a baby, noticed it not breathing properly and started a bag-valve mask until it screamed into life. My hours of neonatal resus training were not in vain.

I realised how much I would miss the team. They were going to be fine without me. But how would I be without them?

I gave Weyni a final hug, we took some more photos and said our last goodbyes. I handed the reins to Jane and a weird feeling came over me, which I can only describe as like giving away a part of myself, forever.

At the airport, waiting for my flight out of Ethiopia, I struck up a conversation with a fellow traveller who told me they used to work for MSF. In the past I would have jumped at the chance to speak to someone who had experience working in international humanitarian aid. And I still do, but now I had my own story to share as well. It felt like an accomplishment.

I remembered the first time I introduced myself as an international humanitarian aid worker – at Istanbul airport on my way to Tajikistan for my first MSF assignment. Then, the words felt chewy coming out of my mouth, like I couldn't quite get them out. Now, the words were there – right on the tip of my tongue, ready to be spoken – but something stopped me from saying them. I held back, and I wasn't entirely sure why. I had something to say, but I couldn't. I was speechless. Silent. What had just happened?

Once more, I was at a crossroad, except the road was an eight-lane highway and I had no idea which direction to go in. Should I take another MSF position to sink my teeth into now that I had some experience? Should I return to Sydney to take James out on a date, if he accepted? Should I do another stint in the Northern Territory and keep working toward being an RFDS nurse? Should I buy a one-way ticket to the North Pole, or settle down in a small cottage in the country? Who knows. All I knew was that I needed to be home in Crookwell for my niece's sixth birthday in July. I couldn't break a promise to a five-year-old.

CHAPTER SEVEN

Back to the Top End

'Careful of the dingos, Miss!'

– A concerned little boy

It was time for my next contract. My friend Jess, a fellow nurse I met in 2009 in Sydney when we were both starting out in our careers, had done locum work in the Northern Territory previously. She spoke to her previous boss and together we accepted a quick three-week contract north of Alice Springs.

The clinic was huge and the team – which I was joining as a nurse, not a midwife – were efficient and reliable. Like all other clinics I'd worked at in the NT, this clinic was established to provide holistic primary healthcare to various communities.

Everyone was super supportive. My first patients were a nanna and two of her grandkids. They all needed seeing to – check-ups and immunisations. It was a full-on morning, but the doctors made sure I had everything I needed to treat the patients properly and efficiently. A far cry from my world in Ethiopia and a nice change of pace to have all the equipment, running water, and a secretary organising an easy flow of patients within time slots.

I lived in a donga, an old shipping container that had been converted into a one-bedroom apartment with a bathroom, kitchen, living area and dining room. I felt like I had space to breathe again. Having spent seven weeks at home living with my parents on the farm, the walls had started to close in on me. Don't get me wrong, I love my hometown and my family, but I needed my space – especially at this time. I hadn't been in a good headspace. Let's rewind …

* * *

After my MSF mission finished, I spent ten days playing tourist and travelling through the north of Ethiopia with my friend and project coordinator Emma, whom I'd worked with in Pugnido and Gambella. We both needed to take a

188

moment – and take a breath – before we re-entered 'the real world'. We did that standing atop the Simien Mountains in the Ethiopian Highlands, watching the sun set over the horizon, alongside the gelada monkeys. On the trip, Emma and I didn't talk about our respective missions, or the future; we were just in the moment together. It was a necessary pause.

We travelled from Lalibela in the Tigray region to visit the exquisite rock churches in the area. One of them was called Maryam Korkor and it was carved into a white sandstone cliff. We were the only tourists there on the day, so we were allowed inside to watch the service. An old nun who lived full time on the mountain was chanting and her voice echoed all around us, sending us to another world. Eventually we came back to reality, and started on the steep trek back down the mountain.

I left Ethiopia for my mandatory debriefing in Berlin. It was there, in the German capital surrounded by familiar items of the Western world, that the true scale and complexity of my time in Ethiopia started to unfold. The debrief wasn't just about giving an update on the mission and providing feedback to the powers above, it was about checking in and emotionally processing the experience. There was plenty to unpack: the trauma, the death, the sheer scale of the refugee crisis. However good the intentions were, it felt very surreal, like a conveyor-belt, ticking-the box situation.

For nine months I had lived on adrenaline, and the moment I stopped, I fell apart.

It started with a toothache. I knew I had to go to the dentist when the pain became so bad that I couldn't enjoy any food in Berlin. Sitting in the dentist's chair, opening my mouth wide for a woman who spoke only German, I felt uncomfortable and vulnerable. I was putting all my faith and trust into someone who I didn't know, who I didn't understand and who I couldn't communicate with. It was an insight into how many of my patients would have felt; with a foreign, English-speaking woman between their legs during such a vulnerable moment of their life. I'm certainly not comparing my toothache to childbirth, but you get the point. My role had been reversed, I was sitting on the other side, and I didn't much like it. Still, being a patient is a reminder of the difference a smile, or a reassuring hand squeeze, or a kind voice can make – even if there is a language barrier.

With my toothache healed, I met my friends Jords, Sam, Tarz and Jess in Georgia for a no-plan adventure holiday complete with good friends, delicious food, a car, hiking and exploration. I then headed west to London to stay with my friend Laura. I was doing what I thought I should be doing: spending time with mates, taking a break and having a good time. On the surface, I was enjoying myself, but underneath that, I was treading water. When Laura went to work, I was alone for the first time in more than nine months. I had no obligations or pressures and soaked up the solitude in her posh apartment. (My definition of 'posh' means it had a flushing toilet, a pantry full of food and carpet.)

For the first week there, I slept, and slept, and slept. One night I slept for eighteen hours straight. I hadn't been through a physical trauma, but it certainly felt like my body was trying to heal itself. I was taking stock. I spent most of my time inside. Being outside on the London streets was overwhelming. The amount of people, noise and movement exhausted me. I couldn't keep up. I forced myself to a daily yoga class, and spent the rest of the time watching new episodes of *Grey's Anatomy*.

Fortunately I had plans to go back to Georgia to meet my soul sister Henriette from Norway – what better therapy than time with your best mate? We soaked in the hammam baths, hiked the Bakuriani Mountains and hired a car and drove to the northern wineries. Henriette describes me during this time as 'still, but not calm'.

I knew it was time to unpack my backpack and return to some version of normality. After nine months in Ethiopia, my debrief in Berlin, a holiday in Georgia, a deep sleep in London and back to Georgia, I headed for the farm.

I made it back for my niece's sixth birthday – arriving in Australia the night before – and the look on her little face was priceless. There were hugs all round. Naturally, I was happy to see everyone after so long away. I was home, but I felt lost.

It was like being trapped between two worlds: the privileged and the impoverished. When I tried to speak about my life in the refugee camps in the Gambella region, I was met with blank stares, or worse, pity. I don't blame people for not knowing how to react to my experiences – heck, I don't even know how to react to a lot of them – but I started to feel like I couldn't speak about them. And I really needed to talk, to be heard and to be understood. I found myself reaching out to friends who worked in humanitarian aid, who could offer their own insights and familiar perspectives and stories.

The realisation that I hadn't hit any societal milestones came to me in fragments. I was helping two of my friends move into their new house when it sank in that I didn't have a home. I was visiting one of my besties in Sydney when she told me she was thirteen weeks pregnant, and my joy for her reminded me how alone I was. One night when I was having drinks with some mates, I couldn't help overhearing a group of younger women near us gushing over an engagement ring. I would try to share a memory from the maternity ward in Tierkidi when someone would change the subject, and I realised that what I was saying was traumatising. Although people wanted to know, they could not relate or share similar stories. I was on the outside of my previous inside world.

I had nothing, only stories. And these stories were hard to hear, they were too intense, too gruesome, too real. I was too much. I didn't fit and hadn't succeeded in fulfilling our society's deemed milestones.

So, I stopped speaking. I didn't become mute, but I stopped talking about the year that was, the things that kept me up at night and anything of importance, and sat back to listen to everyone else. I smiled and nodded and made small talk. Inside I was screaming, but only pleasantries came out. It wasn't just that I was scared of traumatising people, I was scared for myself. If I started talking, I didn't know what would come out. I also didn't know what people would think of it all. Would they think I didn't do enough over in

Ethiopia? That I did the wrong things? That I could've done more or been better or stayed longer?

I was consumed with a sense of guilt. There I was, living in the safety of Australia with my family close by and all the privileges of the Western world. Meanwhile, there are hundreds of thousands of refugees in need of basic medical care, clean water and shelter. And my incredible team in Ethiopia were still working relentlessly to provide a safe place to deliver a baby. My heart ached for them.

'I think Prue's soul is tired,' Mardi said to my mum.

She said what I hadn't yet been able to put into words.

I didn't seem to fit in the world I previously belonged in. The boiling point came when a friend unloaded to me about how stressful it had been picking out new tiles for her bathroom. I know everything is relative – and that we all have our problems – but in the grand scheme of things, bathroom tiles aren't something to stress over. When I bluntly said to her, 'There're people dying in the world, what do tiles matter,' her response included pity, acknowledgement and awkwardness. Where do you take a conversation from there?

* * *

Trauma from my kind of work builds up like a brick wall. One traumatic thing happens, a brick is laid. That brick is solid; it's not going anywhere. Then two weeks later, something else might happen. Another brick is laid. Over time those bricks accumulate and all of a sudden you look up and there's a massive wall. If that wall is too big you can't get over it. So how do you function with this new wall in place? I figured out that I could build around it.

When I returned from Ethiopia there were several walls and I didn't know how to get around them. The reverse culture shock of coming back was so traumatic. I didn't know how I was meant to exist in this world with that knowledge.

I heard about a theory called the circle or ball of grief. If someone in your life dies, you experience a ball of grief. Previously it was thought that the ball gets smaller and smaller over time until you're okay. But now the theory, which I can completely relate to, is that the ball of grief will always be the same size. It will never get smaller. It will never change. It is still going to be this massive hole of sadness and loss and longing. But what happens over time is that you grow around the ball. It doesn't take all of who you are; it doesn't consume you anymore. Somehow I managed to practise this theory to reintegrate back into my world at home.

* * *

I'm not a martyr and I'm certainly not a saint, but it felt like I had been looking at the big picture for nine months while people at home were watching the small screen. It was hard. Instead of talking about what I'd seen – which I really needed to do – I shut down. I stopped speaking because I didn't know what to say.

Everyone has lived and experienced things – I'm not special – but I felt like I was stagnant while everyone else was standing on the green grass and moving forward. I didn't want to feel like this, but I couldn't help it.

Even though it had been nearly a decade since James and I had ended things, I felt I needed to act on my hopes about him. Maybe going back and being with him would solve everything? This was delusional, I know, but somehow I fixated on it and sought him out. After all, we were still mates. And he still hadn't answered my question from the previous year. I was on a mission to find out the answer.

'Hi, I want to see you, when are you free next?' I messaged him.

'What do you want from me?' he replied.

'I want nothing from you, a friend?' That wasn't true. I thought harder and decided I had nothing to lose and everything to gain. 'I told you something true over a year ago. I want an answer. That's honestly what I want.'

'You want something from me, and I can't give it to you,' was his response.

I was devastated and felt like my soul was being crushed. The world I envisioned for myself was evaporating. I'd always said James made me feel like a giddy teenager, but with one message he brought me back to reality. I wasn't a schoolgirl with a crush, I was a 32-year-old woman who'd been holding on to a fantasy for far too long. It was a punch to the gut. Deep down I knew it was coming – I knew I was living in a dream world and putting James on a pedestal – but it still hurt.

In the light of the morning, I still felt sad, but alongside the sadness was a sense of relief. I could move on. I could leave my fantasy in the past – where it probably always belonged – and start to make plans for my future. I didn't hold any harsh feelings toward James. How could I? He didn't do anything wrong. I was the one who had made something out of nothing in my mind.

This was further proof that I needed some help. My adjustment back to the culture I grew up in was harder than I'd expected and I needed help to process this and gain perspective.

* * *

One day Jess and I drove five hours to a remote community. We saw patients for the day, then after closing up the clinic she and I jumped in the car and drove around town to make sure we'd seen everyone who needed to be seen.

We ended the day with a 6-kilometre wander up the road. (There was only one road.) The sun was setting in the distance, painting the sky candy colours, and kids were riding tiny peewee motorbikes. They followed us on our walk and one of them yelled out, 'Hey Miss, careful of the dingos!'

'They're more scared of me,' I shouted back.

'Yeah, but worried about your safety, Miss,' he said. Bless his heart.

We slept in an old house. The dust on the counters told us how long it had been since the clinic staff had visited: it had been a while. We woke up early in the morning to get back to the main clinic. I was glad to be able to get right out into the outback. I felt like I could breathe here. I was doing what I love and reminding myself that I was good at it.

On the five-hour drive back, I chatted to Jess about the state of my life, and she shared her observations about my return. I'd travelled with her in Georgia just after I finished my MSF mission, so she saw me then, and was seeing me now.

'I think you're slowly growing in confidence again,' she said, having noticed how quiet I was when I'd arrived. 'I know it's hard to talk about things, but it's almost your duty to share your stories and to create awareness. We want to hear what you have to say.'

It sounded so easy! I knew I needed to get out of my head and to get things off my chest, but I didn't know how. It was something I needed to work on. But first, patients!

Back at the clinic, I saw back-to-back patients; from a two-month-old baby with respiratory issues, to a 62-year-old also with respiratory issues. The next day, I shared a clinic room with Jess and we did a family immunisation blitz. We treated a nine-month-old baby with impetigo, saw a case of chronic disease of the lower lip, and removed an Implanon from a young woman. Making the tiny incision in the patient's arm, I felt like a real nurse again.

I wasn't on-call so my weekends were my own. What a luxury. I joined Jess and some new friends and we went out to a secret camping spot, where we found an ephemeral lake. It was 5.30 pm when we arrived, so we didn't waste any time jumping into the water for a swim and a play on the paddleboard. It was the start of spring and the temperature was perfect. Not too hot, not too cold, just right, as Goldilocks would say. We lit a campfire, cooked up a feast and, after a few glasses of wine, fell asleep under the stars. *This is living*, was my last thought before I drifted off.

In the morning, we planned to head out on an extended paddleboarding adventure on the lake, but forgot to pack the sunscreen. No bother. We used a local trick and covered ourselves in clay from the bottom of the lake. We must have been quite the sight: a group of visitors, covered in mud, paddling on a fleeting lake.

I was still finding spots of clay behind my ears and on the backs of my knees on the drive back. We stopped in at Banka Banka Station for a stickybeak and then at Threeways Roadhouse for a burger. This was the point where you can go three ways: north to Darwin, south to Adelaide, and east to Mount Isa and Queensland. It's quite the tourist attraction in these parts. The wall of the roadhouse bar is covered in numberplates from the ACT to Alaska. I wondered how they'd all ended up here, at this junction in 'the middle of nowhere'. I wondered how I got here, too.

Sunday rolled into Monday. One week led into another, and before I knew it, I was packing up my donga and saying goodbye. The more I thought about it, the more I understood that the 'middle of nowhere' depended on where you came from.

Before I headed back east, I made a pit stop back in the Red Centre. There's something about this part of Australia that keeps calling me back. The red dirt has gotten under my skin and under my fingernails and up my nose – it gets everywhere. It's a feeling.

It's not just the great group of friends I have or all the happy memories from over the years, there's something about the place itself that draws me back. I know I'm not the only person who feels this connection. I headed out on a hiking track up to a peak on one of the ranges. A black kite watched me from above, as I made my way up the rocky path. The air was clean, crisp and fresh.

At the top of the peak, I took a seat on a rock and admired the view. I'll never get tired of this view: the red dirt, the pockets of green bush and the endless blue sky. 'I love this place,' I thought to myself. Then I had little chat to myself. I was practising using my words, getting them out, vocalising my thoughts. It was easy enough when no-one else was around.

On my way down the range, I ran into a smiley chap on his way up. He struck up a conversation and I noticed a stunning blue pendant around his neck. Before I could ask him about it, he was off, following my footsteps to the peak. Not too long later, he was back. And he was running.

'I didn't realise the time, I've got to get to work. I'm a tour guide out here,' he told me, almost jogging on the spot to keep his momentum.

'Can I take you out for a drink sometime?' he kept talking, and jogging, as he put his number into my phone.

It was a funny interaction, but I didn't think anything of it.

I was talking to my mum on the phone as I walked the last of the track back to the main road. There were rocks and prickles galore, so I was watching my footing when something bright caught my eye. It wasn't a sparkling shard of mica or a red cockatoo feather. It was a colour that belonged in the sky: bright blue. I bent down and picked up the smiley chap's pendant.

I got back to my friend's house where I was staying, and she told me it was a sign from the universe. I sent smiley chap a picture of his lost pendant.

'Wow, thank you,' he wrote back. 'My mum gave it to me for good luck in Alice Springs. Stoked you found it for me. Can I buy you a drink to say thanks?'

The drink would have to wait. I was off on an adventure with some friends to Kings Canyon via Ntaria (Hermannsburg), which sits on the banks of the Lhere Pirnte (Finke River). The Finke is the oldest river in the world – older than the Nile in Egypt and the Susquehanna in the US. The ancient riverbed snakes through the Central Desert Region, bringing water – and life.

From Ntaria, we took a dirt road to Watarrka (Kings Canyon), completing the iconic rim walk, then on to Kings Creek Station to sleep in a swag overnight before getting up to go to Curtin Springs and visit the mighty Uluru. The rock sees you before you see it. It rises from the dirt and holds a captive audience. Standing at the base of Uluru, everyone thinks the same thing, 'Wow, it's big.' Like we all know it's big, but it's really, really big. It takes four hours to walk around it, or three hours on a bike. We opted for the bike ride. It's hard to take in all of Uluru's glory up close, so we also admired it from afar at sunset. Wow, it's big and just captivating.

After another night in the swag under the stars, we hit the road back to Alice Springs and picked up a hitchhiker with a broken bike on the way, exchanging stories and finding out how he ended up in the middle of nowhere on a remote highway with a broken bike, in the heat. He ended up sleeping in my friend's shed overnight and had left for the rest of his adventure the next day.

Over dinner with friends, I pulled out some photos from Ethiopia. It was the first time I'd shown them to anyone. There was the view from the guard tower in Kule with a line of local women carrying heavy bags on their heads. The outlook from the window of the delivery room in the maternity ward we opened in Tierkidi that I spent many hours looking out of. A toddler cautiously inspecting my training doll 'Emilie' at Pugnido Hospital. The toddler wasn't sure of the doll, which looked like a smaller, plastic version of him, but the midwives and incentive staff loved her. Dolls don't exist in that part of the world, so Emilie was a real novelty.

There was also a photo I took at 2 am at Pugnido Hospital while I was leaving after an emergency. The patients had taken their mattresses off the beds and put them on the floor. There were three people sleeping on one mattress on the cold tiles. This wasn't dissimilar to Alice Springs Hospital where carers sleep on mattresses on the floor.

The last photo I showed them was a selfie of me with the premature twins who were brought into the Pugnido clinic weighing just 1.3 kilograms and 1.2 kilograms. That was when I was called in to assess the babies, and I mistook one of them for a pile of cloths. The photo was taken before I transferred them to Gambella. The twins were wrapped up in a blue blanket and I was holding them both in one arm. My smile said it all: 'They're still alive!'

It was nice – and almost a relief – to share some memories from Ethiopia. My friends at dinner were a mix of nurses and their non-medical partners. I spoke freely and they listened. It felt like a step forward in my healing process.

Before I left Alice Springs, I met the smiley chap to return his pendant. He was a lovely bloke, who at thirty-seven had left the corporate ladder behind for a simpler life. He found it – like so many of us do – in the middle of the desert. Over a couple of cold beers, he told me stories of the ridiculous tourists and spectacular sights he'd seen as a tour guide. We had a good laugh together, but even if 'the universe' did bring us together on that hiking track, we would never go anywhere. I was on the move again. This time, I was heading further north.

* * *

I'm not wearing the right shoes. It's a Wednesday afternoon and I'm in a pair of Birkenstock sandals, my happy pants with a loud print, and a singlet. I've been working in the far north. As soon as we get the emergency call-out, my mind goes straight to my feet. Later I find out that during stressful reactions people can focus on irrational items. Mine, it appears, was my shoes.

I don't know exactly what emergency I'm about to face, but I know I'm wearing the wrong attire for it. The local cops called the medical centre for urgent assistance, but they were in too much shock to give a proper debrief on what had happened. All they could tell us was that it was a motor vehicle accident. 'It's bad,' they said.

There's no time to change into a more appropriate outfit. Two cars head out immediately, and I jump in with one of the doctors. We arrive on the scene. And what a scene it is: two groups of people are lying on the road or sitting in the dirt in various states of distress. There's been a serious accident involving a car which has rolled an unknown number of times at speed. The speed, the slippery sand on the side of the corrugated unsealed road and a slight corner created the perfect conditions for a hell of a crash.

We're 26 kilometres out of town, 26 kilometres on a rough, corrugated, dusty dirt track away from the medical clinic. There are five adults and five children all needing medical assistance. The injuries are unknown and the severity unknown. All we can do is our primary assessments, treat what we can, stabilise their cervical spines and get them to the clinic. My default mode was to go into action, based on the mass casualty training I did with MSF in Germany, and managing the training for a mass casualty response in Pugnido.

The cops have managed to get everyone out, and they've started wrapping up the obvious wounds with bandages from the first-aid kit in their patrol vehicle. They've stopped traffic and are controlling the situation. It's all hands on deck. This is the biggest and most serious incident any of us have ever been called out to; the number of people and severity of their injuries is overwhelming. But I don't have time to be overwhelmed. We start doing what needs to be done.

We prioritise the most critical patients and divide and conquer treatments. After our primary assessments, we cannulate people to give them fluids where needed and start to make a plan to get everyone back to the clinic. We haven't got any of the equipment or medication that we need out here. I'm connecting a bag of fluids into a patient, but don't have anything to hold the bag up. I ask a bystander if she can hold it for me.

'Yeah,' she says, walking into the bush and away from the bag I've asked her to hold up. 'Gee thanks,' I think, but before I can come up with a plan B, the woman is back. She's carrying a stick, which she hits into the ground and attaches the fluid bag to. She is a genius.

Because we didn't know the extent of the emergency, we've come into it blind. I grabbed the trauma bag on my way out the door of the clinic, but we didn't bring any analgesia pain medication because it's locked up in the drugs cupboard. Luckily, the doctor finds one vial of morphine in the bottom of her bag. It's not going to go very far here, but it's better than nothing.

Two women are clearly in a lot of pain, crying out. We are careful not to allow their screams to deter us from any more silent serious cases. We clear out the back of one of our troopies and put the back seats down so the women can lie flat. We don't have splints or a spine board, so we stabilise them as best we can. As soon as they're loaded into the vehicle, we tell the driver and a nurse to get them out of here.

'Go, just go. As quick as you can, back to the clinic,' I say, radioing the clinic (there is no reception out here) and updating them on the number of patients incoming. They make the appropriate call to CareFlight (the Top End's equivalent of the RFDS) to attend. There are two CareFlight aircraft on their way, with two pilots, two nurses and two doctors on board.

We set up another car in the same way, and put some walking wounded in the back. They're banged up, but they appear okay. We don't have enough nurses to go around, so an adult family member who happened to stop at the crash site goes with them. 'Go, just go,' becomes our catchcry. We repeat the process until all the patients are on their way to the clinic. Assess, stabilise, go, just go.

I worry about the gentleman with the sore neck. He has a potential c-spine injury. He needs to be lying flat and kept as still as possible to prevent further injury and possible quadriplegia, but we don't have any more vehicles with enough space for that. A man with a troopie pulls up and, although the back is full of building and paint equipment, he offers to take that out, lie the seats flat, put the man in and drive to the clinic.

'As long as the cops can look after the paint,' he says. 'It's my whole work kit for the entire week.'

The cops are happy to mind the paint and the doctor and I jump into the back of the troopie with the man, balancing between ladders and paint tins. Halfway back, we come across the first vehicle that left with the two women, they are not coping on the corrugated road and are screaming out in pain. Analgesia is at the end of this road but they are in too much agony to get there. A quick shuffle of staff and the doctor goes with the two women and the nurse and whatever is left out of that one vial of morphine. Then we all continue in convoy slowly to the clinic.

Everyone is on their way back to the clinic. I don't have time to look in the rear-vision mirror and reflect on what I've just witnessed. If I did, I would have seen blood on the red dirt, drying under the hot afternoon sun. I would have seen a carload of belongings flung into the bushes and beyond. I would have seen the crumpled remnants of a beige Toyota.

Back at the clinic, it is jam-packed. Along with the ten patients, we have the CareFlight medics, our nurses, doctors, and a medically trained visitor who came in when she heard what happened.

'Can you suture?' I ask her.

'Yep.'

'Great, suture that kid up for us,' I delegate, pointing to the young boy covered in cuts and gashes from the broken glass. It takes her two hours to dress all his wounds.

We jump from one patient to another doing primary and secondary assessement, taking blood sugar levels to make sure no-one is hypoglycaemic. We cut off clothes so injuries can be treated. We administer pain medication and start intravenous antibiotics. We have the worst affected three in one room together. The man from the back seat of the painter's troopie is critical, but everyone else is either serious or stable.

We set up a whiteboard with a map of each patient's situation and the plan, including up-to-date information to provide some communication in the chaos. We figure out who needs to be transferred most urgently, who can be sent to the district hospital at Gove and who needs to go to Darwin Hospital. The plan keeps us focused. And we need it. The doctor from CareFlight is struggling with the multitude of injuries. He appears to be in a really heightened state and is working on overdrive, so the whiteboard helps to bring his and everyone else's adrenaline down a level.

The driver is refusing to be seen until his family have been looked after. The wound on his arm was wrapped up with a bandage at the scene, and I convince him he has done everything he can, we are looking after all his family and we have a plan to transfer them all out, but I need to see what's under that bandage and do a secondary survey on him. He finally sits and allows me to assess him. He is running on adrenaline, and so am I.

'Are you in pain?' I ask.

'Nah, nah, I'm right,' he insists.

'Let me just have a look at what's going on under there,' I insist and take him into a treatment room. When I unwrap his bandage, I realise how deep the wound is. It's deep, really deep. The man's entire forearm muscle has been sliced off and the tendons are visible. When the man wiggles his fingers, the tendons dance like puppet strings.

'Oh shit,' I say to myself. Completing my secondary survey I go and update the CareFlight team that we have another surgery case.

The team works together to manage the transfers out, how to get them to the airstrip, who's flying where, and who can wait for the return plane to pick up the remainder of patients.

The first round of transfers includes one of the teenage girls, who's stable but still in a pretty bad way. We suspect she has multiple broken ribs, possibly the clavicle too, but nothing more extreme than that. Her vitals are stable and I get her up and help her walk to the bathroom so she can go to the toilet. She is obviously in pain, but she makes it, insisting she doesn't need any more analgesia.

It's not until they're in the air that the medics realise she has a pneumothorax (collapsed lung). She struggles to breathe mid-flight. The medics are able to do needle decompression and keep her alive on the flight to Darwin. At the hospital there, she's found to have a broken sternum, multiple broken ribs, a lumbar fracture in the spine, a spleen laceration and the pneumothorax discovered on the flight. She's intubated at the hospital and taken straight to surgery.

One of our supposedly least severe patients turned out to be the most extreme. How did we miss that?

With the most critical patients on their way to definitive care, and all the others in a stable condition at the clinic, I take my first deep breath of the day. We take stock of the incident and I feel proud of the work I did alongside the team. We debrief, give praise where it is due and congratulate everyone on their efforts. We then reflect on what we could have improved, what went right and what went wrong.

I can be my own worst enemy in these situations. I tend to focus on what I didn't do, not what I did do, and I don't take compliments well. I am aware of this, but take solace in always knowing I have done the best I can with what I have. The clinic doctor who arrived at the scene with me tells me how impressed she is with how I handled the situation. I thank her for the compliment and credit it all to my MSF training and work.

There is a common criticism of people who go overseas to do humanitarian work: why go to another country when there are so many places here in Australia that need healthcare as well? It's a valid point. Though, I would argue that the skills and lessons I learned on my MSF missions will be a benefit moving forward. The car crash is a prime example of that. Had it not been for my experience working on the frontline in Ethiopia, I wouldn't have been able to handle the crisis in the way I did. Being on the ground and seeing how the medics responded to urgent situations over there is something you can't learn from a textbook or a lecture.

When I get back to my house after the mayhem of the day, the first thing I do is kick off my Birkenstocks.

* * *

The next day, the hauntingly beautiful lyrics of Gurrumul Yunupingu are sneaking through the window from the aged care home next door to the clinic.

It was my first week working here on another RAN contract. My role was on the primary healthcare team with a focus on women's health, specifically testing for, treating and raising awareness of sexually transmitted infections (STIs), and inserting and removing Implanons, depending on the woman's choice. A far cry from the zero contraceptives available in my job in Ethiopia.

I was also feeling temperature whiplash. The air-con in the clinic was blasting. Outside it was 37 degrees and

100 per cent humidity. When I walked out the front, it was like stepping into a sauna. The extreme change in temperature was a shock to my system. In Ethiopia, there was no air-conditioning, so I was just hot and sweaty all the time. The air-con here was a momentary reprieve, a cruel tease.

A call-out forced me out into the heat. A man had been bitten by a dog in the community. I was driving in the troopie on the way to treat him when I heard a story on the radio: a local ranger had been taken by a crocodile, her body had been found a kilometre away from where she went missing, and the croc had been shot. It's all in a day's work in the NT.

Outside of Implanons, I was on-call for any and every medical need. Through the night, I saw a six-year-old boy who'd bitten his tongue and taken a good chunk out of it. Ouch. Then I was called out to an anaphylaxis reaction. The patient had swelling, abdominal cramps, shortness of breath and an alarmingly high respiratory rate. Talking to the on-call doctors, with no planes available we tried to stabilise her with adrenaline, hydrocortisone and Phenergan. After four hours of watching her closely, she was cleared to go home. Still, it was a scary reaction to an unknown cause. I knew that we'd won the battle, but we hadn't yet won the war.

When I arrived there, I felt like I'd chosen the hard (and lonely) road. Now I thought that path was doing me good. I was adapting to life back home and gaining confidence. I'd started to let myself process the magnitude of the last few years. I wasn't shying away from it: the good and the bad. And I wasn't shying away from telling my stories. I bonded with the clinic midwife, Annie, and shared some of my memories from the maternity ward in Tierkidi. Her response was humbling.

'Wow, it's pretty amazing what you were able to achieve over there,' she said.

Instead of downplaying and deflecting my work, I accepted the compliment, I let it sink down under my skin and warm my bones.

In the morning, Annie knocked on my door and woke me up with ice cream for breakfast. I might have arrived there alone, but I wasn't on my own anymore.

At the clinic, I helped Annie with one of her patients: an eighteen-day-old baby who had lost 630 grams since birth. We organised an emergency evacuation flight to take the baby to the nearest hospital. I thought back to my first ever baby evacuation and acknowledged to myself how far I'd come, how much I'd learned and how much I'd grown as a nurse and a person.

On my day off, I went on an adventure with Annie and two other nurses. The word 'magical' gets thrown around too easily, but this place was. The water was so turquoise and bright it almost hurt my eyes to look directly at it. We were the only people there, on this pristine beach surrounded by thick bush. There was nothing manmade in sight, not a building in the distance, a boat on the horizon nor a piece of rubbish on the shore. We were it. But there was a distinct feeling that we were not on our own. I kept an eye on the shallows for any signs of a croc – the lost ranger fresh in my mind – and didn't get too close to the water's edge.

I found a distraction from my loneliness in Annie and the other team members at the clinic. They were an eclectic bunch, ranging in age from twenties to sixties, and they all told engaging and thought-provoking stories. We talked about our travels, previous marriages and relationships, adoption, same-sex partnerships and generational change. They were meaningful conversations, ones that you learn and grow from.

At my next on-call duty, I treated a 31-year-old man experiencing sudden onset severe back pain, and a 54-year-old woman with shortness of breath and chronic obstructive pulmonary disease. I treated both with medication and crawled into bed at 2 am. I cursed myself for spending a day out in the sun prior to an on-call shift. Some things are harder to learn.

* * *

One day by chance I came into contact with a woman called Kate when I was making some phone calls at the clinic.

'Is this Prue Wheelwright?' she asked.

'Yes, it is,' I replied.

'It's Kate, how're you doing?'

I'd met Kate in 2016 and she'd been a remote nursing inspiration, everything she had done I wanted to do. Kate is a realist: she doesn't sugar-coat anything and understands the limits of modern medicine. I distinctly remember Kate telling me a story about her MSF work overseas of shoving premmie babies down her bra to keep them warm and alive, but realising she was only delaying the inevitable. Listening to Kate's stories added fuel to my fire to work internationally with MSF.

Now we were back in touch again and I was able to tell her some of my MSF premmie baby stories. We compared notes before I had to keep on making my calls. It was nice to be in touch again.

After a day in the office, I spent a day doing blood tests, giving medications and reminding people of appointments at the clinic. One lady told me that she was due for her rheumatic heart disease injection. So I went back to the office to check her records and found her again later in the day.

'You have my needle?' she called out to me.

'Yeah,' I said. 'Do you want to go inside to have it?'

'Nah,' she replied, flopping onto a mat on the ground outside and pulling down her undies to show her bum cheek.

'Just do it here.'

'Okay, no worries.' I did as I was told. Her family got a good laugh out of her antics, and I now have that vivid memory.

In my last week on this contract, a gorgeous young girl yelled out to me on the street, 'Hey, pretty lady, where you from?'

'A long way away,' I said.

Immediately, I thought of home. It had been three months since I was last there.

I ran the numbers in my head. In six years I hadn't stayed at the same address for longer than four months. In the three years since I turned thirty, I'd spent thirteen sporadic months at home and twenty-three months away. The time had come.

The road less travelled had taken its toll on me, and even though my work had made me stronger, I needed a rest. I was tired. As Mardi had said, 'my soul was tired'. She was right, of course. I wanted to put down some roots, to have a sense of security in my life – and a postal address. Maybe not forever, but for now.

In the decade since I graduated from university and became a nurse, I'd ticked off so many of my career goals. I'd managed to save up enough money for a house deposit. I'd travelled the world and seen places most people never will. Still, there was something missing. I was sick of changing address and coming back to an empty house. And having to cook for one person. And laughing at my own jokes.

I'd exchanged a few messages with James since the Great Rejection of 2018, and I'd been relieved to feel ... absolutely nothing. The buzz and excitement I once felt when his name flashed up on my phone screen had faded and left behind a simple appreciation for our shared history. I wasn't a giddy schoolgirl anymore, I was a grown woman who could tell the difference between fantasy and reality. It only took a decade.

I remembered a piece of dating advice my godfather gave me: 'Stay in the paddock long enough for the stallions to realise you are there.' I'd been out of the paddock long enough.

I was ready to love and be loved. I wanted to feel at home with someone again – and I wanted to be closer to home.

But before all that …

CHAPTER EIGHT

Queanbeyan

'There's a three-drink limit in the thermal pools.'

– The bartender at the thermal pools, Iceland

D o you ever think to yourself, 'How the hell did I get here?' It's a question I've asked myself plenty of times before, and one I rarely have a straight answer to.

I'm in a steaming hot thermal pool in the faraway mountains of Húsavík, Iceland, looking out over the cliff edge at the ocean below and the snow-capped peaks in the distance. It's 38 degrees in the water and 2 degrees outside. The steam rises to the heavens and flushes my cheeks on the way. The skin on my fingers and toes is wrinkled. I'm sipping a glass of champagne with my lifelong friend Andy and shaking my head in amazement. There's a yellow lighthouse on the horizon and from afar it looks like a friendly dinosaur. At this point it wouldn't surprise me; this place is surreal. Also we're a little bit drunk; there's a reason for the three-drink limit in the thermal pools – it goes straight to your head.

How did I get here? Technically, I flew fourteen hours from Sydney to Doha, another eight hours to Edinburgh and two and a half hours to Iceland. Logically, I booked a ticket to the World Extreme Medicine Conference in Scotland with my paramedic friend, Andy. We had come this far; why not extend our adventure to a road trip around Iceland, in search of the aurora borealis?

The best of the best in remote healthcare was at the conference, and I was ready to learn as much as I could from them. Doctors and nurses spoke, and there were also talks by NASA astronauts and aquanauts (yes, that's a real job), survivors of the 2015 Mount Everest earthquake, ocean rowers and Bhutan critical care helicopter pilots. This was medicine at its most remote and austere, from ice to dirt, the skies to the seas.

On the first day of the conference, I attended a talk by a Canadian remote flight doctor. I saw myself in his stories: the nurse on the ground, waiting desperately for help to land on a remote airstrip. Day two was all about humanitarian work, so once again I saw myself reflected in the stories. Many of the speakers had worked with MSF, and were leaders in safety, security, communication and rehabilitation in disaster settings. I met so many incredible people and heard so many extraordinary tales. It was inspiring, exhausting and a little intimidating, but I felt like I belonged. I'd earned my stripes. I'd done the work and now, seeing so many other avenues that work could take me, I was excited.

Talking to many women, I find they they are like me, very quick to feel like an impostor. We're conditioned to be humble, polite and self-deprecating. We're expected to play down our achievements and bat away compliments. There have been many moments in my life when I've felt out of my depth. I know I'm good at my job, but I still feel like an impostor, which I don't think is a bad thing. It's what keeps me going, to work hard to be constantly learning and to be able to say when I don't know something.

I think of my grandma Mardi, one of the few women working in the male-dominated physiotherapy field in the 1980s, and how she would have had to back herself every single day, every single time she walked into a meeting room, every single moment she spent dealing with bigoted clients who mistook her for the secretary. I think of how far women have come since then, and how far we still have left to go.

On the last day of the conference, I participated in a simulated terrorist attack. There were smoke machines, (blank) gun fire and actors made up like they were victims, covered in blood. It was all very realistic and overwhelming. I went into autopilot mode and got the job done the best way I knew how. I still have a lot to learn and I was invigorated by the experience and the teachers. At the end of the simulation, I came out the other side feeling exhilarated. And also pretty exhausted.

I went to the pub for a steak dinner with Andy and we reminisced about our trip so far. We'd gone from exploring glaciers and staying in homely B&Bs, to responding to a fictional terrorist attack dripping in fake blood. The difference between Iceland and Scotland had been noticeable, going from a blissful holiday to a working holiday. Staying with Emma, my friend from Pugnido, we explored the city of Scotland and beyond, hiring a car and driving as far north as the Isle of Skye. We fell in love with the scenery, and the accommodation was exquisite – as Andy described it, a place where 'the showers made love to you, and the beds hugged you'. We had a great trip.

A week earlier I had been admiring the force of Dettifoss, the second most powerful waterfall in Europe, and swimming between the tectonic plates in the cold, pristine Icelandic water of the Silfra. A single week before that I was rubbing aloe vera cream into my sunburn from the stifling sun of the Top End, and in a week's time, I would be at home, dipping sheep with my dad on the farm. Oh, what a difference a week makes. I liked to move but it was time to stand still.

* * *

The person in my life who sees me the most clearly is Mardi. She has this phenomenal ability to know the right questions to ask to get me to open up and face the truth (even if I haven't figured out what that truth is yet). She also has an innate ability to listen to what is not being said, listening to the silence in between. It's my first Christmas at home in five years and I'm relishing my time with Mardi and the rest of the family. But underneath the Christmas cheer, I'm feeling lost and angry.

'I have no idea what I'm doing,' I confess to Mardi.

'No-one does, darling, no-one does,' she reassures me.

It's such a cliché to reassess your life and goals at the end of the year, and that's exactly what I'm doing. I'm fortunate to have the time and space to be able to do that, back here, in the family home I grew up in.

'I'm so happy to have you home,' my mum says repeatedly, pulling me into a warm hug. 'Sorry it's so quiet!'

'Mum, I need quiet,' I say wholeheartedly.

Having spent the better part of a decade in far-flung places, I've been craving 'quiet'. I don't want adventure or adrenaline when I'm home, I want to stop. I want to help Mum clean the windows and do a puzzle with Dad. I want to walk into the pub and know everyone there. I want to breathe in the familiar fresh air that takes me straight back to my childhood.

More than anything, I want to buy a cushion. No, seriously, I have this overwhelming urge to buy a really nice cushion. But in order to have somewhere to put the cushion, I need a couch, and for that I need a room, and for that I need a house – you get the picture. I feel a deep desire to put my roots down and buy a house, and for that I need a mortgage, and it turns out the banks are not super enthusiastic about lending to a contract humanitarian aid worker. So I need a full-time job.

On New Year's Eve, I resolved to make 2019 my year of balance. A year of no travel. To stay put. Do not leave the country. I'd poured myself into working and travelling, and now I needed to focus on finding some stability, and hopefully some love. The psychologist I started seeing explained it perfectly: 'A chair has four legs. So does life: family/love, career, community, and social/leisure activities. If the four legs aren't the same height, the chair is going to wobble.' My chair is so uneven, I'm about to fall off it.

In 2012, I visited a witch doctor in Livingstonia, Malawi, on a trip through Africa. The man had drooping earlobes, piercings all over his face and an eccentric energy. He ate hot coal and predicted my future. Sitting on a decorative carpet, the witch doctor told me that by age thirty I would be married, have four kids, I would still love my job and I would live in England. Sure, it was probably a well-rehearsed tourist trap, but still … I didn't want to disappoint the witch doctor, so I set out to tick off some more predictions. Better late than never, eh.

Queanbeyan

*'You've always been a lucky child, because you
were born with a fairy looking over you.'*

– Grandma Mardi

I was in the back of an ambulance, holding my patient's hand. The 23-year-old woman presented to Queanbeyan District Hospital at thirty weeks pregnant, concerned about a decrease in foetal movements. Her patient records told me this was her first pregnancy. I took her blood pressure and it was 160/110, which was dangerously high. I tested her urine and found protein. I determined that she had pre-eclampsia, and she and her baby were at risk. The woman was terrified as we organised her transfer to Canberra Hospital. Although it was extremely unusual for a midwife to be taken off the ward and sent on a transfer, the paramedics were not comfortable with the situation, so I opted to escort her.

The Queanbeyan District Hospital wasn't set up to deal with cases of thirty-week deliveries, so the safer place for this woman and her unborn child was the Canberra Hospital, which was a twenty-minute drive away. For the woman, it felt like the longest drive of her life. For me, it was a luxury compared to the four-hour trek from Pugnido to Gambella Hospital, or organising a plane to some remote area to take a patient to the closest hospital.

The woman was silent, but her face spoke volumes. Her furrowed brow showed her worry, her upward glance told me she was pleading with a higher power in her mind, and her tight grip on my hand said she was clinging on to hope.

I looked out the windscreen and spotted the sign for the Canberra Hospital. It was only when we pulled up that I let go of the patient's hand. There were red marks on my palm where the woman's fingernails were digging into my skin. I took her inside the (enormous) hospital with the paramedics, and trusted that she'd be in safe hands. On our way out, the paramedics offered to give me a lift back to Queanbeyan, so I jumped into the back again.

We made it out of the hospital and around the corner before the paramedics were called to another emergency. A 72-year-old man was experiencing shortness of breath and chest pains. The sirens blasted, the lights flashed and the driver put her foot down. I held on. I was here for the ride.

When we got to the patient, the paramedics went into battle mode. The man was having a heart attack and needed to get to hospital immediately. I helped to insert a cannula in the patient's arm and then waved them off. From the side of the road, I called the Queanbeyan Hospital and told them my location. Which was interesting as I had no idea where I was. I'd just moved to the area. One of the community nurses came to pick me up and take me back to finish my shift.

It was my first day working at Queanbeyan District Hospital, which was a typical regional community hospital with 140 beds and a close-knit team. Everyone knew each other: from the cleaners to the kitchen staff, doctors to receptionists, and paramedics. My role was full time, and the idea was for me to work across both the maternity ward and emergency department. It was the best of both worlds for me; the joy of delivering babies and the challenge of facing emergencies. As much as I was happy to be on home turf again, I couldn't help feeling like I was taking a step backward. After doing challenging placements out bush and overseas, I was back working near home.

Queanbeyan is an hour and a half south of where I grew up in Crookwell, and it has a country town charm even though technically it's a part of Greater Canberra. There's a Kmart here, but fifteen minutes away in downtown Canberra there's a Myer, a sushi train and a major tertiary hospital.

I surprised myself and settled in quickly to life in Queanbeyan, and enjoyed the work. It was a full house on my afternoon shift – with three midwives we had nine patients and babies in a seven-bed ward – and I was in my element. At 5 pm, my patient in labour started to progress with the help of some gas. She was screaming, cursing and hitting the roof when she delivered a beautiful baby boy. At 7 pm, my 42-year-old patient was silent and composed as she delivered a baby girl. Then, at 9.30 pm, a woman was transitioning and, although my shift was meant to finish at 10 pm, I stayed on, and at 10.25 pm the woman delivered a baby girl.

There's no such thing as a textbook birth. Every birthing experience is different. Some women scream, others stay silent. There's no 'right way' to have a baby. It's about empowerment and a belief that we are capable. The only thing that's been consistent, in all the hundreds of births I've witnessed as a midwife, is that women are incredible. Women are made for this; medicine should only intervene if required. However, in our current world it seems we are taking a massive leap toward an intervention-heavy medical model of obstetric care.

At this well-resourced regional hospital, I had access to equipment and technology that I could only dream of in Ethiopia where I'd once used a stray clean razor to cut a cord. And yet, there were still challenges. Here in this modern hospital the cord is cut with single-use sterile metal scissors which are discarded afterwards. The waste does not go unnoticed. How useful those scissors would have been in Ethiopia. Other challenges were largely ego-driven and probably due to having too much access to too much intervention. There was a doctor who trained in ED but had transferred to obstetrics. In ED, doctors are go-go-go, but in the maternity ward, things run at their own pace. A lot of our work is having the ability to sit and wait. This overbearing and interventionist doctor wasn't used to not being in control, and tried to push things to happen on their own schedule. I struggled with that. All my training, experience and instincts had taught me to take a hands-off approach, so it was hard for me to work alongside someone who was hellbent on doing the opposite.

Our profession is sadly changing for the worse; it has become over-medicalised, standardised and overly structured. It no longer seems to focus on the normal, but how to make the normal complicated. It doesn't focus on the individual's wants, needs, culture, beliefs or desires, instead it puts them in a medical system that seems to disregard the normal progression of labour and birth, starting the clock once they arrive at hospital.

However there is the 'midwifery model of care', which is based on the fact that the pregnancy and birth are a normal and natural part of life. This approach puts the woman first; their wellbeing is at the centre of care. Midwives monitor the physical and psychological health of the mother and provide her with education, choice, counselling and hands-on support throughout her pregnancy, labour and birth and post-partum period. This model of care minimises technological interventions and has been proven to reduce birth injuries, trauma and unnecessary c-sections. Sadly, these models are fading away and there is not enough of them in Australia, herding women into a health system that overmedicalises something that is completely normal.

* * *

Outside of work I moved in with my cousin Jen in Queanbeyan. Conveniently living one block from the hospital, I was doing what I set out to do for the first time in a long time. I had a regular social life. I was doing a weekly park run with a group of people, catching up with mates for steak at the pub on a Wednesday night, and opening myself up to the world of online dating.

I was also visiting the family farm, or meeting Mum for breakfast halfway, and spending as much time with Mardi as I could. My fierce grandma at this stage was living in a nursing home in Crookwell. She was as sharp as ever mentally, however growing increasingly forgetful and, concerningly, she was declining physically. Her body was giving up. She was losing strength and mobility. That's often what happens in nursing homes. When you don't need to cook for yourself or walk to the other side of the house to go to the bathroom, you lose those skills.

Mardi's trademark ferocity was still there, but there was a fragility as well. It was painful for me to see, but more painful for me not to. On a visit, she told me something profound. 'You've always been a lucky child, because you were born with a fairy looking over you,' she said. I smiled. Maybe she wasn't completely there.

I talked to Mardi about the house I was looking at buying. 'It's a two-bedroom place on a quiet street, with high ceilings, two bathrooms, a garage, a courtyard with a deck, and it backs on to a nature reserve,' I told her, brimming with excitement.

'Prue, I can't walk up stairs!' she said.

'Don't worry, we'll carry you,' I replied. I couldn't wait for Mardi to visit me in my own home.

The closest I'd come to owning a home was buying a tent. I was excited about having my own place, somewhere I could hammer nails into the walls and paint the door blue, or red, or whatever colour I wanted. I spent too much money on paint samples and two hours in the tile section at Bunnings. Remember a year ago when I rolled my eyes about my friend complaining about how difficult it was picking the right tiles? Yeah, I'm a total hypocrite. Look at me now.

The joy of marking a milestone was only slightly tainted by the thought of having a thirty-year mortgage and being tied down forever, but that was something I was working on with my psychologist.

Truthfully, I don't think I would have gone to see a psychologist if it had been left up to me. Thankfully, the MSF end of mission package covered a certain number of sessions. I figured I might as well use some. As much as I told myself I was okay when I got home, I wasn't. That was a hard thing for me to admit. No-one likes being vulnerable.

I don't think there's any shame in seeking help for mental health issues, but it's still not an easy thing to do. There's this stigma that if you see a psychologist there must be something wrong with you. It's total bullshit. If you break a bone, you should see a doctor. In the same way, if you break down, you should see a doctor. There is no easy diagnosis and fix for mental health problems.

There's a power in admitting you're not okay, and in realising that it's okay to not be okay. Struggling with mental health doesn't make you weak or lesser than, it makes you human. I think medical professionals are expected to have a tougher skin, but everyone needs help no matter how strong they appear.

I had a breakthrough with my psychologist about the enormous pressure I put on myself to do it all and be it all. He told me I needed to change the way I set goals for myself. Goals are never-ending. Once you reach one, there's always another and another. After getting my nursing degree, there was a midwifery degree. After finishing my first RAN placement, there were two more and then MSF. After MSF, there was a giant hole.

My psychologist taught me to stop chasing goals so that I could tick them off and add another to the list, and to instead enjoy the ride. Reaching goals doesn't necessarily make you happy, so you have to make the most of the moments on the way. It sounds so simple, but it was a big lesson for me.

* * *

I was on the phone to Mum when we got the news: Mardi had a fall at her nursing home in Crookwell and was on her way to Goulburn Hospital. Shit!!! I told Mum I would ring the hospital when Mardi got there to see what the situation was. 'She's not talking, is quite confused and is bleeding a lot,' they told me. I jumped straight in my car and set off on the hour-long trip to Goulburn. I was concerned, but I tried not to stress. Old people have falls, this happens, I saw it all the time.

At the hospital front desk, the receptionist told me that Mardi was in Resus One, the most critical bed. This was where patients were taken if they needed life-saving treatment immediately. I started to seriously stress and just wanted to get to her.

When I was finally allowed in to see Mardi, I was horrified. Walking to the side of her bed, I realised she had no idea who I was. Her eyes were vacant. She didn't recognise me. I thought, 'The person who has always seen me for who I truly am can no longer see me.'

It was a split-second moment, a bolt of realisation, and it shattered my heart to pieces. I swallowed hard and blinked fast to keep my tears from spilling. I didn't want Mardi to see the pain on my face. I switched into nurse mode and helped the hospital nurses to roll Mardi over and gently wiped the blood off her. Once she'd been cleaned up and seen to, I held her hand and talked to her. But grief took over and I burst into tears. Mardi didn't flinch. She didn't know who I was, what was happening, or why I was crying uncontrollably. Once the tears came, they didn't stop. I had to remind myself I was not her nurse, I was her grandchild. Being at a patient's bedside as a loved one was not a role I liked playing. It also dawned on me that all those frail elderly people who come into hospital have a story. They have a family; they have decades of stories to tell and memories to share. They should be the most valued members of our community, yet we lock them away in nursing homes to wait for their demise.

When I eventually had to leave the hospital, I went home, where Mum and Dad were waiting up for me. It was after midnight when I pulled into the driveway and crumbled into their arms. My grandma, my mentor, my biggest inspiration in life and my biggest cheerleader, was gone. She was still alive, but she was gone. There was no coming back from this.

The next day we were advised that Mardi had two bleeds on the brain, and the prognosis was uncertain. We were told that she could stay the same as she was last night (unable to communicate or recognise her loved ones), or she could improve, or she could die. The unknown was scary.

After a week in Goulburn Hospital, Mardi was transferred back to Crookwell, and we made sure she was comfortable and not in any pain. The hope was that she would fall asleep peacefully and not wake up. I think that's the hope we all have, isn't it? For the life to be long and the death to be quick.

You'd think seeing death on a regular basis at work would make it easier. It's not. Sure, I understand that it's a part of life and we're all going to die one day, but that understanding was cold comfort when I saw the shell of my grandma in a lounge chair in a nursing home absent-mindedly watching daytime TV.

While Mardi was fading away from us, I was working my regular shifts in emergency at Queanbeyan Hospital. Work was a distraction I needed. In the ED, there was plenty to think about. I started my shift at 1 pm. A 73-year-old presented with heart attack-like symptoms, and we assessed, diagnosed and treated him appropriately. An eight-year-old girl came in with diabetic ketoacidosis. We inserted two intraosseous needles and started life-saving treatment on her, and escalated the case to Canberra Hospital. I finished my shift at eight o'clock the next morning, nineteen hours after I started it.

The ED was a mixed bag of all sorts. There were a lot of mental health cases. Because of the scale of the issue, systemic failings and society's tendency to not take mental illness seriously, people slipped through the cracks. I saw it happen first-hand.

A man presented to the Queanbeyan ED with suicidal thoughts. 'Something's not right, I just need some help,' he said. He wasn't a danger to others, but he was to himself. He'd done all the right things by realising he needed help and seeking it. I admitted him as a high-risk patient and told him he would be seen by the mental health team as soon as possible. I'm not a psych so I couldn't treat him myself. I watched this patient – who had vulnerably admitted to being unwell – sit and wait, and wait, and wait. He was in the ED for five hours before he gave up and slunk out the door. I didn't see him leave, but when I realised he was gone, I was overcome with rage. The system had failed this man, and many more like him. It was a disgrace. For the umpteenth time, I was angry at the health system.

On another shift on another day, I stuffed up. A patient stumbled in covered in grazes. He'd come off his mountain bike and was scratched up, but he was breathing well, didn't appear to be in a great amount of pain and his observations were within the normal ranges. I suspected a broken rib, so I triaged him a Category Four (the second lowest category). He declined analgesia. I organised an x-ray. It was a very standard case, until it wasn't.

I was seeing another patient when the in-charge doctor came up to me. 'You know your Cat Four? He's got a flailing chest.'

Shit.

The patient had broken so many ribs, his rib cage had collapsed and was threatening to puncture his lungs. I kicked myself for not picking it up on admission, but the doctor came to my defence.

'We all would've missed it, you couldn't have known,' he said.

The patient was transported to the Canberra Hospital for management, and he came out the other side fine. I took my negligence personally but also am aware we can't know it all, we can only do the best we can. No harm was done. But still it was a lesson learned and a jab to my confidence.

I was wrong to think Queanbeyan Hospital might be a step backward in my career. The team were incredibly tight-knit, knowledgeable and experienced. I was learning lots of new things and keeping my skills sharp. In the ED, I rotated between triage, resus and team leading. In the maternity ward, I delivered a 2.4-kilogram baby two hours and sixteen minutes after her nineteen-year-old mother went into labour.

I was ticking all the boxes I drew for myself on New Year's Eve: a good job, a mortgage and a house of my own, a social life, and a bloke. I'd started seeing a man named Rob. He was kind, generous and a carpenter (which comes in handy when you're renovating a house). He was the first and last person I met on the dating app a friend downloaded for me. We hit it off and things moved quickly.

I fell in love with Rob's family as much as him. He had lived a very different life to mine, and still lived in his own glorious bubble full of routine, stability, family dinners and hard work. I tried to mimic this bubble and fit in next to him, and his family. He was like a silver platter of everything I'd been looking for, and he wanted the same things as me: a partner in life and a family.

I got what I wanted, and yet still, something was missing. I should have been ecstatic, and I was trying very hard to convince myself that I was. How lucky was I to have everything I wanted. This was what I wanted, right?

I remembered what my psychologist said about goals: they only lead to more goals, enjoy the now.

I wondered if I was settling because I was afraid of being alone. Then I wondered if I was running away because I was afraid of commitment. I weighed it up. Is it better to be with someone who doesn't see you for who you really are? Or is it better to be alone, staring at yourself in the mirror?

I didn't know the answer.

I wanted to ask Mardi, but I couldn't. She was gone. On 8 April 2020 – six months after her fall – she took her last breath. It was an enormous loss, but also a relief. Mardi never recovered from her fall, so even though we lost her, she'd already been gone for a long time.

In life, Mardi left a huge mark on me. In death, she leaves an empty hole.

CHAPTER NINE

Back to the Red Centre

'You need to find the balance between giving
and receiving.'

– A good friend

Sunshine is standing in the doorway, refusing to move. There's no other way to get into the house. I try reasoning with him, but he doesn't listen. He sighs and turns away, pointing his rear at me. Sunshine is a giant chestnut horse.

I'm two and a half hours drive from Alice Springs on a mostly sealed road. On the way into the community, we come across horses and donkeys on the track. I'm sure the horse that was on the track and wouldn't move out of the way of the troopie must be a relative of Sunshine's. There are a lot of stubborn horses, cheeky donkeys and 200 people with four RANs running the clinic. This place feels like a little oasis nestled among the MacDonnell Ranges. I'm here for a four-week RAN contract.

This wasn't part of the plan. I was meant to be growing roots and settling into my home in Queanbeyan with my partner, Rob. But the Red Centre and RAN autonomy called, and I answered. I even agreed to a two-week Covid quarantine in Alice Springs prior to going out remote.

I arrived on a winter's afternoon and tried to get my bearings. After a tour of the medical clinic – including introductions to the team and the resident cat – my new manager pointed me in the direction of the valley. As instructed, I headed off for a walk as the sun started to dip. The ranges were glowing, and brumbies galloped in the distance. I drank in the postcard-worthy scenery. Glug, glug, glug.

My first day in the clinic started with a fifty-year-old woman complaining of pain 'down there'. It was the first time she'd had pain like this, so she was worried. I examined her and prescribed the necessary treatment.

My second patient was a shy, young woman, who didn't make eye-contact with me and mumbled her words. After repeating herself a few times, I figured out that she wanted her Implanon removed and a new one reinserted in her other arm. The first one had been put in three weeks ago and it was hurting her.

The day ended with a planned non-emergency evacuation to Alice Springs Hospital. A local woman had a severe kidney infection and needed treatment, so she was being flown to Alice Springs. While we were at it, I was given a tour of the airstrip. It was a hell of an airstrip – the fanciest I'd seen – surrounded by the ranges, with a long stretch of dirt and a huge pest-proof fence all the way around it. There was no need to turn the troopie high beams on here and do laps of the runway to scare the roos off. One, because of the fence, and two, because planes weren't allowed to land here at night. The mountain ranges are too difficult to navigate in the dark. If there was an emergency overnight, we either had to take the patient halfway to Alice Springs by road to pass them over to an ambulance, or drive them to the nearest airstrip to hand the patient over.

On my first night of on-call duty, I prayed that I didn't have to do an emergency evacuation. I didn't. I saw a kid at 8 pm with a possible dislocated shoulder, and another child at 10 pm with a cough. I got a full night of uninterrupted sleep in my house, a seven-minute walk from the clinic.

On Saturday, I climbed to the top of the helipad. It's not a real helipad, rather the slang name of a peak on the edge of town. It's a steep thirty-minute walk to the top and a slippery scramble down. My legs burned on the walk back to my donga, but it was a good burn.

In town, I saw Sunshine being tormented by some dogs, so I shooed them away and led him out of trouble. I felt sorry for him, so I opened up the garage door at my accommodation to give him some hay I had seen there previously. But I made a foolish mistake: I didn't realise Sunshine was right behind me. When he spotted the hay, it was game over. He charged into the garage and started devouring the hay. I tried everything to get him to move outside, but it was impossible, so I moved the hay instead. I ended up with a laundry full of hay and a very overfed horse.

With the remaining hay safely behind closed doors, Sunshine eventually trotted off. I swear I saw him smirk.

How was I going to explain this to my manager? It was her hay.

* * *

I've added a new skill to my arsenal of RAN tricks: cigarette rolling. It's beneath tea making, porridge cooking and medication coaxing. It was my first time visiting a palliative care patient, who asked me to roll him a cigarette (something I had never done). It was a sloppy job, but he didn't seem to notice or mind. He was one of four patients the clinic did daily home visits to. As well as rolling him a cigarette, I made him breakfast and made sure he was comfortable.

Next on the list was an elderly woman who was given medication; a thirteen-year-old who needed insulin and meds; and a mental health patient who required his daily anti-psychotic medication.

On my way back to the clinic, I ran into my first patient here – the fifty-year-old woman – and she gave me a big smile. The medication was working.

It was a big day: the optometrists were in town for their annual visit, a big undertaking since we were in the midst of Covid and its restrictions. I helped the two young women set up; eight patients came in, and eight patients went out with a new pair of glasses. I finished my shift and told the optometrists to come and find me if they needed anything. 'My house is the one with the ambulance outside,' I said. 'You can't miss it.'

The next morning I headed to the clinic to start my shift while the optometrists were packing up their car. I'd said they could go into my place if they needed to and an hour later, I got sent a photo. It was of Sunshine inside my lounge room. The enormous horse filled the whole room. He had snuck into my house after I left for work and while the optometrists were distracted outside. They managed to coax him out with some food, but not before taking some happy snaps. What an eventful trip for them.

At home after my shift, I got a different kind of visit from a group of kids. They were a curious bunch and I invited them in for some frozen mango and oranges. They walked around my house, checking things out with orange fruit peel smiles. They left with some oranges for later, and I told them not to let the cheeky horse in on the way out.

It's incredible how quickly I felt like I'd slipped back into community life. I couldn't imagine for a second having a horse in my lounge room in Queanbeyan, but here, it was just another day at the office. I had a whole life waiting for me in Queanbeyan – a house, a stable job and a boyfriend – but it felt so far away from here and now. It felt so far away from me. I had thought I wanted stability and normalcy, but now that I had it, I felt like I was losing a part of myself.

I felt more alone in that world then I did out here where I was truly alone.

I wrote an expression of interest to the Royal Flying Doctor Service. I didn't know if I would send it, but it felt good putting it down on paper. Was I really looking at escaping what I thought I wanted and dreamed about? Hadn't my past mistakes in leaving a relationship for work opportunities taught me anything?

The winter rain swept through the desert and brought new life with it. In this moment, the grass was quite literally greener out here.

Greener, but also dirtier. I washed the clinic troopie that ran patients to and from Alice Springs Hospital and the dirt from the outside of the vehicle muddied the ground. Inside, I found old chicken bones from KFC (I hoped), chips, lollies, melted chocolate and sticky patches of spilt fizzy drink (I hoped). It took half a day to clean, and I doubted it would stay clean for long.

* * *

In this line of work, I see life at its beginning; I nurse a six-day-old newborn.

I see life at its end; I help transport an elderly patient from the community where he's lived his whole life to palliative care where he will spend his final days. I try to advocate for him to stay home and pass away. But his family did not choose this option.

And sometimes I see life before it has a chance to begin. A patient comes into the clinic. She's ten weeks pregnant and is experiencing abdominal pain and bleeding. I assess her, explain the likelihood of a miscarriage, prescribe her pain medication, and tell her to come back if things get worse. She does come back, and things do get worse. She is miscarrying and there's not much we can do other than make her feel comfortable and supported. Depending on how the miscarriage progresses, we might need to transfer her to Alice Springs for a dilation and curettage to clear the uterine lining, removing any leftover tissue to prevent heavy bleeding and infection. It's hard to know how this patient feels, she is expressionless and silent. It is not my job to tell my patients what to do, I am here to give them information and support so that they can make the right choice for themselves. I am also here to hold their hand when they are scared.

My patient is so much more than a statistic. At the clinic, we make small talk and find out we have the same birthday.

We were born on the same day in the same year and have found ourselves in the same place at the same time, for very different reasons.

Soon it was time to make some decisions for my own future. I hit send on the expression of interest I wrote to the RFDS.

* * *

During a weekend in Alice Springs I talked to my friends about my life back home, the pull I felt for there, the fact that I was lost. They joked that I was always lost. Everything I thought I wanted was waiting for me back home, including the newly renovated house full of cushions. We brainstormed, ran through what-ifs, drank many bottles of wine and tried to find a reason why I felt so ill at ease. I spoke to friends from all over who appeared to be happily married, asking how they knew, whether they had any doubts, what was it about their partner that made them decide to commit the rest of their life to them. I spoke to my family who had welcomed Rob and adored him, spoke of my trepidations, my feelings, my doubt. I didn't know what I was looking for; some clarity, maybe, some direction, someone to tell me what to do. But of course no-one could make this decision for me, I had to make it myself.

I tried everything to change myself, to make myself happy with choosing a life with Rob. I pondered over the weekend's conversations on my way back to the clinic for the last week of my placement. Inside, my mind and my heart were torn.

I heard back from the team at the RFDS and they pencilled in a video call with me. I figured it would be an informal chat, so I didn't get my hopes up, but the thought of working for them stirred something deep inside me. It would be my absolute dream job, combining all my passions: maternity, emergency work, community and travel.

I was working on the day of the RFDS call, so I took my break to have 'the chat'. Except the chat was a fully fledged interview. When I logged on to the video conference, there was a panel of three people waiting for me. They asked big questions – 'What frustrates you most in your line of work?' – and specific ones – 'How would you handle a case of pre-eclampsia in community?' Even though I hadn't prepared for an official job interview, I felt good about my answers. Especially when they asked me, 'Why do you want to work for RFDS?' I'd had five years since my first airstrip experience with the RFDS to think about all the reasons I wanted to be on that side of the emergency.

The information they gave me added even more reasons to my list. First, they told me the starting salary, which was higher than I was expecting. Then they told me that after six to twelve months experience, there was the possibility of working nine weeks on and nine weeks off, which would be entirely liberating. When the call ended, I felt like I finally knew what I wanted, like I had something important to work toward, like there was something for me to hold on to when I blew up my life.

I had made the decision; I needed to end things with Rob. He wasn't the person for me, even though I was trying desperately to make it work. It was a tough call to make, and a tougher conversation to have.

Queanbeyan, 2020

'You're a unicorn.'

– My gynaecologist

We had the conversation soon after my return to Queanbeyan. there were tears, and an almost-proposal. When Rob professed his love for me and dropped down to one knee, I told him to get up. 'Don't ask that question because you know the answer,' I said. 'You can't do that to me, I can't do that to you.' Over time, through talking to his family and through kindness and honesty, we both came to terms with it. He moved out of the house, and it ended with a lit candle and a note left on my kitchen bench.

'The final chapter has come to an end. What a journey it has been. I will always remember us as two people who fell in love on our first date. I accept your heart's decision that I'm not the one. Let this candle shine. When you blow the flames out, this will be the final chapter closed,' the note from Rob read.

With hesitation but clarity, a sense of certainty and a tear, I blew out the candle. I knew I'd made the right decision, but that didn't make it any easier. Walking away from Rob also meant taking steps away from my hope of becoming a mother and having a family. I turned thirty-five soon after, single and with a new, surprisingly fierce ovary scream that was demanding children. I know how fickle fertility is, so I booked in to see an obstetrician-gynaecologist who specialised in fertility and IVF. I was trying to take some control. If I decided I wanted a baby, did I have the physical, emotional and physical means? Would I have my family's support to do it alone if I decided to? I was heeding the scream from my ovaries, exploring the options.

The first step on the journey was the standard gynaecological consult. When I was younger and had a Mirena IUD inserted, the doctor did an ultrasound and told me I had a bicornuate uterus (a heart-shaped uterus). She assured me it was only a slight one and that it wouldn't affect my ability to have kids. I hadn't thought of it again until this moment when I gave my gynaecologist my medical history.

She booked me in for an internal ultrasound. Later that week when I attended, the ultrasonographer left the room and came back with the head of gynaecology at the clinic. My dear friend Tarz was with me, and I made eye-contact with her. 'Oh shit,' I said.

It's never a good thing when they bring the big guns in. I know the signs: hushed tones, sympathetic eyes, uncomfortable body language. I was about to get bad news.

'You have a unicornuate uterus, Prue,' the gyno told me. 'You're a unicorn!'

As a midwife, I knew what that meant. As a patient, I had no idea what that meant.

'Basically, the uterus is meant to be a three-bedroom house. Yours is a studio apartment,' the gyno explained. 'There's still a chance you'll be able to conceive, but it's more complicated. You have a higher chance of miscarriage, stillbirth, premature birth and ectopic pregnancy.'

It's a rare condition – one in 4000, I was told – and I was born with it.

The diagnosis was a blow. I spent a lot of time researching and processing. I found plenty of positive unicornuate uterus stories: women who made it to thirty-six weeks in their pregnancy, mothers who only discovered they had the condition after they gave birth. Although the risks were higher, it wouldn't be impossible for me to have a healthy pregnancy. I decided I wasn't going to let my unicornuate uterus stop me from having a child if I decided I wanted one. Also I came to terms with the fact that there's more than one way to become a mother.

For the first time in my life, I started to picture what a life without kids might look like. I'd always wanted to be a mum – it's such an expected thing for women – and I just assumed it would happen when the time was right. I felt like I'd been climbing a mountain – building a career, searching for a partner, making a home – and trekking toward a peak.

For me, that peak had been entangled with being a mother, birthing a child and raising it. Now, as I'd grown, I'd spotted an entirely different peak on another mountain in the distance. On this peak I was not a mother. I felt like I would have missed out on something on this new mountain peak. But I realised that even though this peak had a different view, it was wonderful, full of possibilities and dreams not yet had. It was full of the magical powers of the unknown. Maybe, in fact, I was coming to terms with not being a biological mother.

CHAPTER TEN

The Royal Flying Doctor Service

'Don't forget to breathe.'

– An RFDS pilot

I've seen Royal Flying Doctor Service planes cutting through clouds in the sky. I've seen them land on red dirt airstrips. I've seen them from the outside looking up, but I've never seen inside them. Until today.

In a word, the inside of an RFDS Pilatus PC-12 plane is: cramped. In two words, it's: very cramped. There are two seats in the cockpit for the pilot. And in the back, there are two stretchers for patients and three seats for the nurse, a doctor and any escorts. There are about 25 centimetres between the nurse's seat and the stretcher. It's a tight squeeze. Every inch of the plane's compartments is full of life-saving equipment and medications. As a newly employed RFDS flight nurse, it's my job to know where every single bandage, oxygen mask and needle is.

I need to have muscle memory when I reach for things in the plane cabin. More than anything, I need to have adaptability. Being an RFDS flight nurse is unlike any other position. We work autonomously yet with all the equipment and experts a phone call away. We need to know what we're doing. There's an added level of common sense, logistical thinking and capability required to do this job. It is not for everyone, even if they have all the right qualifications and training.

I clearly remember the feeling of being a new RAN, nervously waiting for the RFDS plane to pick up my seriously ill neonate patient from the red dirt airstrip. I remember the pure relief of hearing the plane engines in the distance, and the awe I felt watching the medics take over. Being on the other side now is a humbling experience. I'm the person who is going to the rescue, not the one waiting to be rescued.

In order to work for the RFDS I had to do six months of training in intensive care so I could become familiar with how ventilators work, among other things. I first tried to do the training at Canberra Hospital, because I was living in Queanbeyan. I was told that I needed to have worked there for five years before I could even *see* a ventilator.

I then rang the nurse unit manager of ICU at Alice Springs Hospital; I knew him from when I'd worked there previously.

I asked him if I could come and get some ICU experience, as I needed it to work for the RFDS.

His reply: 'When do you want to start?'

So suddenly I moved back to Alice Springs, which felt odd; I didn't think I would be back here. Yet here I was. I had tried the settling-down thing with Rob and the house and then that all imploded because it was just not who I was.

When I arrived in Alice I thought, *Why am I back here? This place is hard. It's very remote. It's so expensive to get out of. It's away from my family.* But then I remembered: I just love it. There's something about it. There's something about the feeling of it. Something about the soul, the earth.

It actually felt right to be back there. I was really happy. Then I went to the ICU and it was a domain I had no idea about, with sick people on huge infusions to keep them sedated and a ventilator that's breathing for them and all of a sudden I had to learn about the mechanisms that in ED I'd had some exposure to, except every time we'd only have the patient for 10 minutes before we sent them off to the ICUs.

It was so interesting learning about the infusions, the lines, the different access points, equipment and things like that. On my third shift I was given a ventilated patient because we were short-staffed. They knew I would ask for help if I was unsure of anything. Also, often the best way to learn is to jump right in. This is my style of learning and I was enjoying the challenge.

I did that for six months and I was still talking to the RFDS, who were saying, 'We're figuring out the start dates. You're doing everything we've asked you to do. Let's get you started.' Then one of the educators told me that I had to do a Critical Care course in Adelaide, at Flinders University.

Some of my ICU colleagues were doing this course and they were in the midst of horrible assignments and exams, spending every other day studying. I did not want to do that at all. What they were learning is down to the cellular level of how stuff works: if you pull out potassium, what happens to the sodium levels, that kind of thing. I'm just not that way inclined. I really wish I was, but I'm not.

Since I had to do the course to work for the RFDS, I made a plan. I did one subject at a time, nice and slowly, to ease my way through. But by this point I knew I would never be an ICU nurse. There's a line of thought that you're either ICU or you're not. You're either ED or you're not. You can't be both. ICU is very particular and very meticulous and organised, whereas ED is just chaos. If you take an ICU person to ED, they generally hate it. If you take an ED person to ICU they think, *This is pretty quiet and a bit too clean. And I've got one patient, what is happening? No one's screaming at me!*

I started doing the critical care ICU component and the first subject was awful. It was looking at the cellular level of a kidney. I was not enjoying the course at all.

So I went back to the RFDS educator and asked if I could go across to the ED component, still at Flinders University. On further questioning I found that that it was just a *preference* for me to do the Critical Care course over the ED course.

That changed everything. I switched over to the ED course and they took credit from the one subject I'd already done in Critical Care, which meant I only needed to do three more subjects. ED was so much more my game. I understood it. We looked at critical care patients, blood results and ECGs. They really homed in on the actual practical stuff that I could see and touch and visualise. Not the cellular count of how the muscle tissue expands in the heart.

Separate to the course, I understand now why the ICU experience was so important – that's because fundamentally what we have in the RFDS is an ICU bed on the plane. Knowing how all those lines work, cannulas and infusions, knowing that meticulous positioning of putting lines into people, that's so important.

During the time I was working in ICU I would meet up with the RFDS managers of Alice Springs central operations and talk about when would be a practical time to start. They asked me how I was going with the training. Although I verbally had the job, I hadn't signed anything yet and I really wanted to sign something to make it real!

* * *

I want to say that boarding my first RFDS flight as a nurse felt like fulfilling my destiny, but actually it felt like any other first day of a new job: eyes wide open and excited about the possibilities. Sure, there was a satisfaction in doing a job I'd always wanted to do and had worked hard to get, but it was still a job. That's been an interesting realisation. So much of my identity is wrapped up in my career, but there's so much more to life than work.

The RFDS team based in Alice Springs with me is made up of high achievers and adventure seekers. The manager remembers seeing my résumé come through way back when I first reached out six years ago after the late-night emergency rescue. One of the pilots, Shane, flew to that case way back then and now I'm flying with him. It's such a kick to join their ranks.

My RFDS medical training was held in Adelaide over two weeks. We spent the bulk of that time doing a general medical refresh, a cardiac crash course and the standard hand-washing credentials, and at the very end of our last day, we got to go on an actual RFDS plane. The other trainees and I did an emergency evacuation simulation, where we kicked out the plane window and climbed out onto the wing. For a job that's predominantly done on a plane, I thought there might have been some more plane training. But, hey, there's nothing like being thrown in at the deep end.

After the training, and back in Alice Springs, I started out doing buddy flights so I could learn by watching my colleagues. I took note of where they put the rubbish bin, how they packed the storage compartments and how they strapped themselves and patients in for take-off. I clocked how they wrangled three patients at once, how they managed their paperwork and what they did when people got airsick. Nursing on the ground is one thing; nursing in the air is a whole other game.

I soaked it all up, and after a fortnight of buddy flights, I was deemed competent to fly solo on a Friday morning. By that afternoon, I was on my very first solo flight. It was a short trip from Alice Springs airport to Hermannsburg to pick up a pregnant patient and transfer her to hospital. It was just the pilot and me. There wasn't a doctor on board. Doctors are not on every flight; they only come when deemed necessary.

It was a simple, standard flight – just eighteen minutes there and another eighteen back – but I was frazzled. The flight was so short, I didn't have time to finish my paperwork. I couldn't figure out how to pull out the stretcher on my own, so I had to ask the pilot for help. I hadn't perfectly memorised where everything was, so things took me longer than they should. It was a sharp learning curve: this was the reality of not having a safety net or a colleague to lean on. The autonomy of being a flight nurse was unlike any other role I'd had. In an emergency department or refugee camp

I had colleagues to work with, to learn and pick up skills from – and vice versa. Here, it's just little old me. On my lonesome. Doing my best.

When we landed back in Alice Springs and successfully offloaded the patient, I felt like a kid in a lolly shop. I was on a high. I did it! I completed my very first solo flight and lived to tell the tale. So did everyone else. Phew.

The RFDS (Central Operations) covers an enormous chunk of the Northern Territory and South Australia. Our slogan is: 'The furthest corner, the finest of care'. The Central Operations team runs four aeromedical bases in Adelaide, Alice Springs, Darwin and Port Augusta, as well as three remote primary healthcare facilities in Andamooka, Marla and Marree in outback South Australia. Every day we assist around 100 patients, be it an aeromedical evacuation, a GP and community health nurse clinic, a telehealth call, a mental health or oral health clinic, or a child's immunisation. I am one of fourteen full-time registered nurse/midwives working in Alice Springs, the centre of Australia's outback. We fly as far north as Elliott (762 kilometres out of Alice Springs) for emergencies, all the way to Darwin and Adelaide for planned transfers, through to the APY Lands in South Australia and across to Kiwirrkurra in Western Australia.

Mostly we meet our patients on the airstrip, but we also go into the nearest clinics to stabilise unwell patients prior to transport. I do love the variety and teamwork of coming together out in the middle of nowhere all for one cause – to keep the patient and everyone else safe. One morning, we can pick up a renal patient needing urgent transport to the hospital (because they've missed their life-saving dialysis appointments since they can't afford the petrol to drive to town and are now profoundly unwell). In the afternoon, we can pick up a tourist who's fallen off a Segway on a tour at Uluru and broken their tibia.

Many of our call-outs are for mental health patients.

Some things never change. I'm still frustrated by the state of the mental health system, just like I was when I was working in Queanbeyan. Mental health affects us all, from country towns to metropolitan cities to communities in the desert. It doesn't discriminate.

* * *

On a regular night-duty shift for the RFDS we went up to Elliott in the Barkly region to pick up a woman who had an infection, but we didn't know where. She was clinically stable and needed to come in for investigation.

I was on my way out to the plane to get ready for take-off when the RAN rang with an updated set of observations. The patient was actually turning septic and her blood pressure was dropping. This is not a good situation.

I was told to wait for the doctor, who was one of my favourite colleagues. Once he emerged, we took off and by the time we arrived, the patient was deteriorating pretty rapidly and I was so thankful the doctor was with me. If I'd been on my own I would have done everything I could do for her, but having him there meant we had a second pair of hands. We worked hard the whole way back to Alice Springs to keep her stable.

When we landed we were exhausted and thought we were done for the night. By then it was about two o'clock in the morning. We were immediately pinged again for another task – an urgent transfer from Alice Springs Hospital to Darwin. The patient was a 21-year-old man who'd come off a waterski at one of the stations. He'd broken his tibia in the fall, then a CT scan showed that his popliteal artery had fully occluded, which meant he had no blood flow to his lower limb. This is very dangerous, and he needed surgery urgently. There was nothing we could do for him on the plane, even though his foot was turning white from the lack of blood flow – he needed surgery when he arrived in Darwin.

After a three-and-a-half-hour flight, it was 6 am when we landed in Darwin. The patient was transported to hospital, but the RFDS team couldn't go anywhere: the pilot had run out of hours and wasn't allowed to fly. Our plane had to stay on the tarmac and we had to stay in Darwin until he was allowed to fly again – for at least ten hours.

The RFDS booked us in for two nights' accommodation at a hotel, because if you check in at 6 am and check out at 4.30 pm you have to book in for the night before and the night ahead.

First we all went out for breakfast. The pilot and the doctor went to bed, but I was wired and awake. I love Darwin. I have friends here, including Jess, and the markets were on. I called Jess and said, 'I'm out the front of your house!' I then helped myself to some of her clothes, a swimming costume, sunglasses and a toothbrush, so I could at least clean my teeth.

We went for a swim, went to the markets and had a lovely lunch. I spent all day with her then went back to the hotel and had a few beers – there was time to kill, after all.

Once the doctor emerged from his room I asked if he'd like to have a beer with me.

He said, 'Well, Prue, like you, I'm about to sit on a plane for three and a half hours and drinking makes me need to pee.' By this time I'd had three beers myself; I'd completely disregarded the three-and-a-half-hour trip and there's no loo on the RFDS plane.

From that point on I stopped drinking everything, including water, before we got back on the plane at about six o'clock that night. My manager had covered my next shift for that night, and by the time we got back it was 9.30 pm and I'd been awake for about 36 hours.

* * *

Let me state the obvious: nursing isn't glamorous. There's blood, vomit, urine and faeces. But one thing I wasn't prepared for was transporting Covid-positive patients from remote Indigenous communities to isolation hotels in Alice Springs. Because, unfortunately, the Northern Territory's efforts to stop the spread to these vulnerable areas were not successful. Fortunately, however, the roll-out of vaccinations in these areas dramatically reduced the mortality and morbidity rate. Transporting the patients in 40-degree heat in the height of an outback Australian summer in full hazmat suits and N95 masks was intense. I thought I knew hot, I was wrong. We sat on ice packs to cool down.

There are many stories, some good, some bad, and some just comical. One day I'm transferring a beautiful old man from Alice Springs Hospital to Adelaide. He is in the grips of dementia and he reminds me of the vulnerability of Mardi in her final days. These are the patients that hit close to home. I want to give them the best care, because that's what I wanted for Mardi, because that's what we all deserve at the end of the line.

This patient is obsessed with having a TravelJohn on him at all times, a wee bag essentially that solidifies liquids to prevent spills. I try to take it off him, but he's not having a bar of it. He clutches his TravelJohn tightly in his hands as we stretcher him into the plane. I walk around the plane to the door, wave off the paramedics who dropped the patient off for us, and when I get on the plane, the man is trying, unsuccessfully, to put the tip of his penis into the TravelJohn. He did tell me he needed to wee.

It happens in slow motion, and there's nothing I can do to stop it. I don't have gloves on, so I reach helplessly for anything to act as a barrier. The pilot in the front is oblivious to what's happening in the back and has locked all the doors for take-off. I'm trapped. There is no way the man is going to be able to aim into the hole of the TravelJohn. Once he starts, it's game over. He covers himself and the plane in urine.

I'm thankful that the man is well-hydrated so his wee is diluted and not smelly. I'm also thankful that it lands in little puddles all over the plane, instead of one giant pool that could seep down into the engine cavity and cause damage. Lastly, I'm thankful I am at his head end, and only my hands get urine on them.

The man is unaware of what's happened, and it's impossible to be upset with him. All I can do is let out a little laugh. When shit hits the fan – or urine sprays the ceiling – you have to find the humour in it.

After take-off when the plane is cruising, I start to wipe up the puddles and splatters. The flight time from Alice Springs to Adelaide is three and a half hours. It's a long three and a half hours before I get to wash my hands properly.

We work on a rotating 24-hour roster. When we're scheduled on, we work a combination of shifts, from restocking the plane and hangar, to picking up clean laundry and pharmacy items, to attending emergency call-outs and completing interhospital transfer flights. We regularly transport patients from Alice Springs Hospital to Adelaide Hospital for cardio stents, neuro management, preterm pregnancies and other cases that Alice Springs Hospital isn't equipped to handle. It's up to a seven-hour round trip in the air and work on either side and in the middle makes for a big day.

On downtime during the longer flights, I listen to audiobooks, study my course books and run through hypothetical situations with the pilot. 'What if I lose consciousness at 20,000 feet?' the pilot quizzes me.

'Well, first I would slap you and wake you up,' I say cheekily.

'No, first you have to breathe. Don't forget to breathe,' the pilot says seriously.

I spend as much time in the cockpit as I can, trying to familiarise myself with it, in the unlikely event that I do have to take control of the plane with my nonexistent flight training. It's a terrifying thought.

When I'm on night duty, I can be at home, waiting for a job to come through. When the inevitable happens, we need to make it to the plane and be ready to take flight in one hour or less. I can be cooking a stir-fry one minute and rushing to treat a neonate who can't breathe the next. Things can change in an instant. Living on standby can be jarring, but my four-month on-call stint in Ethiopia prepared me for this, as well as all the hours spent on-call as a RAN. There's still a lot of running on adrenaline.

I was on a forty-minute flight to a community en route to a Category Four patient who missed dialysis and needed to be taken to Alice Springs Hospital. When we arrived and met the RAN team at the airstrip, the patient was sitting in the front of the troopie, on two litres of oxygen, talking normally and appearing stable. He jumped out of the vehicle and onto the stretcher with ease to be loaded onto the plane. In the time it took for me to hook him up to a monitor and oxygen and to close the plane door, our walking-talking Cat Four patient became a menacing, disoriented mess. He refused to lie down, ripped his monitor off and started removing his clothes. He was panicking because he was struggling to breathe. I was trying to calm him down, but it was no use. His oxygen was going down and his blood pressure going up. It took me a long time to get a blood pressure reading because he wouldn't stop moving and was tangled up in his oxygen cords. We were at the end of the runway ready to take off, but I told the pilot to taxi back to where the RANs were still waiting. Thankfully, it's procedure for the transporting RANs to wait for the plane to take off before leaving. This is the reason why.

I swung open the plane door and called out for help. The RANs climbed on board under the pitch-black night sky and helped me to calm the patient down so we could insert another cannula and give him more medication to settle him and his blood pressure. There were three of us in the back working on the patient, but we couldn't control him. We administered another round of meds, and eventually the man tired himself out from hyperventilating and trying to get naked. I thanked my lucky stars that the patient escalated while we were still on land with help nearby and not in the air when I was all on my own.

As it happened, the patient had acute pulmonary oedema, meaning his heart was pumping too fast and not efficiently enough and his lungs were being filled with fluid so he couldn't breathe. It's not a good situation to be in. To deal with the life-threatening fluid build-up, we needed to force air into his lungs to push the fluid out; but on this nurse-only flight, we didn't have the equipment to do that. We bring that equipment for when a doctor is on board. All I could do was keep his blood pressure controlled until we got to the hospital and keep the bag-valve mask close by in case he stopped breathing.

When we landed at the Alice Springs airport, a doctor, fellow flight nurse and paramedics were waiting and ready to intubate the patient if necessary. I jumped in the back of the ambulance with the doctor and, with lights and sirens blaring, we successfully delivered the patient to the emergency department. My experienced flight nurse colleague followed behind to pick me up and take me back to the hangar. I was in a heightened state and was grateful for his kind words of comfort and compliments. I was focusing on all I did wrong and what I could have done better. As I've said, I am my own worst enemy.

This wasn't an unusual situation in the wild world of the RFDS. The week before, my colleague picked up two patients, one with sepsis on heart medication, and the other had given birth seven hours earlier in community and was being transferred to Alice Springs Hospital for a standard check-up for her and the baby. The woman had had a straightforward delivery without complications and was sitting on the stretcher in the back of the plane holding her newborn. In the air, the mother had a massive post-partum haemorrhage and required three blood transfusions at the hospital. She nearly died. From take-off to landing, things can escalate dramatically, and we need to be prepared for the worst (as best we can in the confines of a tiny plane mid-flight).

Working for the RFDS gives me a newfound appreciation for RANs. Having been on the other side, I know how stressful and challenging working as a RAN can be. On this side, I know the difference a capable RAN can make in an emergency situation. I also have the advantage of knowing a lot of the RANs I run into. One day a RAN asked where he knew me from.

'You're so familiar to me, where do I know you from?' he said.

We both had a think, but I wasn't sure if we had met before. It wasn't until I was preparing to leave that he remembered.

'Oi, you're the RAN from that big car crash?' he said, referring to the ten-person motor vehicle accident I attended. He had driven one of the vehicles from the crash back to the clinic. 'You were a busy lady that day!'

It's a small world out here. I remember the story my dad tells of me looking at the world map on the flight home from Bali and marvelling at how big the world is. How can something be so big and so small all at once? I'll never know.

* * *

It was 2 am. I was on night duty again when we got called out to a patient. A fifteen-year-old kid was 'acting really weird'. The notes explained that the patient couldn't be taken to Alice Springs by car (even though it's only an hour and a half drive) because of his odd behaviour. So, we were sent by air to get him. It was ridiculous. 'As if they can't get a fifteen-year-old, sixty-kilo kid into a car, instead of making us fly out there,' I thought. 'It's probably just a stoned kid acting out.'

It was very early, and I was a little cranky (can you tell?), but we rushed out to the patient. There was me, the pilot and a doctor named Mark. I love working with Mark because he's always so calm and in control and has a wicked sense of humour. He only escalates things when they need to be escalated.

We didn't know it yet, but things were about to escalate. When we arrived we went to the clinic with our trauma kits and found the patient was, indeed, acting really weirdly. He was completely disassociative and not cognitively present. It was almost as though he was having seizures, without the fits. His eyes were opening spontaneously, he was confused, making incomprehensible sounds, and was hitting his head on the side of the bed. He was unsafe to transfer. The kid needed to be intubated. It was my first bush intubation and I was nervous, but it went semi-smoothly, and we transferred the patient to the plane with an adult escort because he was underage. The escort was a massive mountain of a human.

'I'm sorry I'm so big, I don't want to be in the way, but this is my little uncle, so I need to be with him,' he said. He was the definition of a gentle giant.

During the flight, we kept trying to understand what was happening to the patient. 'Yeah, he's been smoking some ganja [cannabis], but that's it,' his companion swore.

The patient was intubated for two days. Bloods were drawn and CTs were taken, but all the tests came back normal. The case was chalked up to being a drug-induced psychotic event from some bad synthetic-laced drugs.

It was an intense case, and another lesson in expecting the unexpected. Always.

I still haven't mastered the art of being hydrated but dehydrating myself for flights, so I was squeezing my bladder tight on an empty flight back to the hangar after a patient drop-off in Adelaide. I crossed my legs tight and thought dry thoughts. As soon as we landed, I rushed to the bathroom, but an emergency was unfolding on the plane landing behind us.

On my way to the bathroom, the pilot of the plane that had just landed after ours yelled out, 'Baby, baby, baby!' I rushed over and found my colleague and fellow RFDS nurse Carol kneeling on the back of the plane between the patient's legs, giving life-saving breaths to a premature baby via a bag-valve mask. Sure enough, a baby had been born seconds before on the tarmac. The mother was only thirty-two weeks pregnant and when the baby boy came out, he wasn't breathing. I jumped into the plane with Carol and Gwyn, the doctor. They were simultaneously clamping and cutting the umbilical cord and resuscitating the baby. Thankfully another experienced nurse/midwife, Jacqui, joined us – we were all crammed into a tight space. We did what we could there and then made our way to the patient transport facility (PTF) in the hangar. Normally, the PTF is empty because the ambulance service is so quick, but today there were three patients sitting around drinking tea, waiting to be transferred to hospital.

In the middle of the room, we pushed the contents off a bench, lay down a towel and continued resuscitating the baby. We needed help so called for a paediatrician from the hospital. Gwyn and Carol had the resus covered, I rushed back to the plane to help Jacqui and the mother. The placenta was out but she had started to bleed, heavily. When it rains, it pours. Getting her off the plane was a priority, so blood didn't seep down into the plane cavity, requiring the plane to be grounded for intense cleaning.

In the bathroom at the PTF, we were treating and cleaning up the mother and sighing with relief when the bleeding stopped. On the bench outside, the doctor was breathing for the baby. In the corner, our three waiting patients had stopped drinking their tea and were watching in shock. When the ambulance and paediatrician arrived, we transferred them all to the hospital.

It was only when the two of them were safely on the road and out of sight that I remembered I needed to wee.

Three days later, I saw the mother and her baby son in the neonatal unit at the hospital. They were both alive and stable. I was overjoyed to see them, and I said as much to the mum.

'Thank you for everything you did,' she said to me, with a shy smile.

'You're welcome,' I said, remembering the chaos.

* * *

I used to joke that being a midwife was my birth control; that every time I saw a third-degree tear from the vagina to the anus, I would delay having a baby for another year. But deep down it was something that I wanted – not the third-degree tear, but the experience of carrying and delivering a baby. I've witnessed the miracle of birth, but I haven't been through it myself. I used to dream about my ideal birth; who my midwives would be and how I would surrender my body and try for as little intervention as possible. I'm now coming to accept that my dream may remain just that: a dream, not a reality. I don't joke about midwifery being my birth control anymore.

In the same way, I don't ask women when they're going to have a baby. It's such a brutal question to be asked, especially if you're struggling with fertility, have experienced a loss, are undecided about having kids, don't want them or simply don't want to talk about your reproductive system. I have friends who have tried for years and spent thousands of dollars on IVF and are still in the trenches hoping to fall pregnant. I also have friends who are happily child-free. I have friends who dreamed of having a boy and a girl and those dreams have come true. The more I start to consider a life without children, the more I notice how many women I know who have chosen the same. I also notice how content, fulfilled and whole they are. There's this idea that we need to procreate to have a purpose, that we need to have kids to leave a legacy, that being a mum is a requirement.

I'm still trying to figure out what my 'purpose' in life is. Mardi never had kids of her own, but she left an undeniable impact on the world and passed away surrounded by the love of her family. Maybe we don't need a 'purpose' and we just need to live. To have good days and bad days and everything in between. To do the best we can with what we have and, above all else, be kind.

All I know is I am only thirty-seven and my life has got a long way to go. There are many stones unturned and obstacles to overcome. Who knows where my life will end up. I know there is still time for me to find a partner and have a child, if we both decide that's what we want, but I'm not waiting on it. I'm living. I'm making peace with the likelihood that I might not become a biological mum, and that has been such a liberating experience. For years I've been focused on listening to the ticking of my biological clock, but now I've tuned it out, I can hear the world around me again. I can hear the cockatoos singing in the ghost gums, I can hear my friend laughing in my backyard, I can hear the rain falling on the tin roof. As for finding a partner to navigate this world, a quote from a friend rings clear. 'The best thing about having your heart broken is the chance to fall in love again.' How nice it will be to fall in love again. One of life's precious gifts.

Through all my stories and experience and fighting and working hard, I have now signed that liberating RFDS contract of nine weeks on and nine weeks off. I feel elated about the unknown and the possibilities to be had in nine weeks off. Imagine that. The options are endless. I can do RAN contract work, possibly another MSF project, go on dates and spend time doing things I love that aren't related to medicine. I know I love to dance, so why not go to Argentina just to dance in the street as I once did? I love to cook, so I'll travel the world doing cooking courses and come home to throw a lavish feast for my friends and family. I love to scuba dive, so I'll spend time in the underwater world every chance I get. But mostly I love travel and being in nature, and what better way to explore that than by doing multi-day hikes, plus there are many, many mountains to climb and countries to explore. The possibilities are endless – who knows what I'll find.

* * *

I'm looking out the window of the RFDS plane, on a flight transporting a 21-year-old woman and her unwell newborn baby back to Alice Springs. This isn't an emergency flight, but it's an emotional one, because the patient's partner had recently committed suicide. Her family had gathered at the airstrip to say goodbye to her. In the pitch-black darkness, I can't see them, but I can hear them talking and wishing the young mother well before we take off.

Out of the plane window after take-off, I can see stars above and below. Except they're not stars below, they're the flashlights on the phones of the family gathered below, being waved in the air. It's a beautiful sight. The pilot, the patient and I turn on our phone flashlights and wave back at them.

This story ends at the beginning.

Under the dark desert sky, an RFDS plane is flying above a red dirt airstrip in the outback. This time, I'm on the plane.

Acknowledgements

Writing a book was never on my agenda; for one, I can't spell. I just passed English at school and despised writing essays for university. Writing is not a skill set I have. But through a series of events, being open to new opportunity and being the 'yes' woman I am, I have landed here, with a published memoir of my story to date. I do not feel special in telling my story, as alongside me are countless extraordinarily inspiring people whose stories all deserve to be told. So, on reflection, why I even have an acknowledgements section in a book is to acknowledge all those who do not have the opportunity to tell their story, to those whose stories fill these pages. And I hope to inspire those medics out there to say YES, to work hard and get out of their comfort zones.

These stories are told from my perspective taken from years of journalling on how I felt at that time. My perspective and opinions evolve as I grow and learn. It is not my intention to cause insult or harm in the retelling of any events in this book.

Where does one start when finding the words to thank everyone? My family, first and foremost I thank you. My ever-supporting mum and dad. Not a day goes by that I am not thankful for having you in my life. Even when I hated you I loved you. Thank you for pushing me and making me who I am today. To dearest Mardi, ironically in your final years I was trying to get you to write a book, because your story needed to be told. Alas, it died with you. I hope this makes you proud. I miss you. To the amazing community and extended family at home who welcome me constantly and support me in all I do: Alex and Jess, Allan and Jo, Lib and Tim, Libby and Ian, Chris and Mark, Laura and Will. To Richard and Jackie for the neverending gin supply and overseas adventures. To my friends who come from near and far, who cover all corners of the globe, I love you all. To my past loves, I do not tell this story to embarrass you or win you back, I'm telling it from my perspective and hope I have not caused you any distress.

Annie and Ben, my home away from home, with countless pick-ups and drop-offs to Sydney airport, a warm bed and delicious meal in between, I thank you. To the countless life-altering moments of joy shared with strangers, from a simple smile to a kind word, acknowledging that we are all humans doing our best with what we have.

To everyone who made this book possible – particularly James Knight and Pip Kensit, who were the instigators and first thread of this book existing. To the wonderful team at Hachette, Sophie Hamley, Jacquie Brown and all in between. Thank you, for seeing something I didn't, and guiding me through publishing a book – a rare opportunity I couldn't pass up. And most importantly, to Alley Pascoe. I entrusted you with my journals, gave my soul on paper to a stranger and took a leap of faith. You are incredible at what you do and the fact that you were able to read my writing and pull together years of ramblings that were never intended to be re-read is indescribable. I thank you.

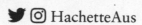
hachette
AUSTRALIA

If you would like to find out more about
Hachette Australia, our authors, upcoming events
and new releases, you can visit our website or our
social media channels:

hachette.com.au

 HachetteAustralia

  HachetteAus